DIAGNOSTIC PROBLEMS IN TUMOR PATHOLOGY SERIES

DIAGNOSTIC PROBLEMS IN TUMORS OF GASTROINTESTINAL TRACT: SELECTED TOPICS

DIAGNOSTIC PROBLEMS IN TUMOR PATHOLOGY SERIES

Series Editors

Arun Chitale, MD (Path)
Diplomate American Board of Pathology (1969)
Surgical Pathologist Sir HN Hospital, Jaslok Hospital,
Surgical Pathology Center
Formerly Professor & Head Department of Pathology Bombay Hospital Institute of Medical Sciences, Mumbai, India

Dhananjay Chitale, MD (Path) DNB
Diplomate American Board of Pathology
Division Head, Molecular Pathology & Genomic Medicine,
Senior Staff Surgical Pathologist
Director, Tissue Biorepostiroy
Assistant Clinical Professor, Wayne State University School of Medicine
Henry Ford Hospital, Detroit, Michigan, USA

Diagnostic Problems in Tumors of Head and Neck: Selected Topics, 1/e
Arun Chitale, Dhananjay Chitale, 2014

Diagnostic Problems in Tumors of Gastrointestinal Tract: Selected Topics, 1/e
Arun Chitale, Dhananjay Chitale, 2014

Published by Arun Chitale & Dhananjay Chitale

Copyright © 2014 Chitale publications

DIAGNOSTIC PROBLEMS IN TUMOR PATHOLOGY SERIES

DIAGNOSTIC PROBLEMS IN TUMORS OF GASTROINTESTINAL TRACT: SELECTED TOPICS

Authors

Arun Chitale, MD (Path)

Diplomate American Board of Pathology (1969)

Surgical Pathologist Sir HN Hospital, Jaslok Hospital,

Surgical Pathology Center

Formerly Professor & Head Department of Pathology Bombay Hospital Institute of Medical Sciences, Mumbai, India

Dhananjay Chitale, MD (Path) DNB

Diplomate American Board of Pathology

Division Head, Molecular Pathology & Genomic Medicine,

Senior Staff Surgical Pathologist

Director, Tissue Biorepostiroy

Assistant Clinical Professor, Wayne State University School of Medicine

Henry Ford Hospital, Detroit, Michigan, USA

Table of Content

PREFACE: VII
Polyps of Gastrointestinal Tract 1
    Introduction 1
    Polyps of Stomach 2
        Hyperplastic Polyp: 2
        Fundic Gland Polyp (FGP): 4
        Definition: 4
        Adenomatous Polyp (Gastric adenoma): 5
    Polyps of Small Intestines 7
        Brunner Gland Adenoma: 7
        Inflammatory Fibroid Polyp: 8
    Colorectal Polyps 10
        Adenomatous Polyp 11
        Serrated Polyps 15
        Hyperplastic Polyp (HP) 16
        Are Hyperplastic polyps related to the genesis of colorectal cancer? 16
        Sessile Serrated Polyp (SSP) Without Dysplasia 17
        Sessile Serrated Adenoma 18
        Villous Adenoma 19
    Miscellaneous Polypoid Lesions 21
        Colitis cystica profunda 21
        Granular cell tumor 22
        Ganglioneuroma 23
        Kaposi's sarcoma of GI tract: 24
        Gastrointestinal Polyposis Syndromes 25
    Heredity and Cololrectal Cancer 25
        Classification of Hereditary GI polyposis Syndromes (Genes), inheritance 25
        Familial adenomatous polyposis 25
        Hamartomatous polyposis 26
        Familial Adenomatous Polyposis [FAP] 27
        Desmoid tumors in FAP 28
        Attenuated FAP (AFAP) 29
        Gardner's Syndrome 29
        Turcot's Syndrome 29
        Peutz-Jeghers Syndrome (PJS) 29
        Juvenile Polyposis Syndrome (JPS) 32
        Hereditary Non-polyposis Colorectal Cancer (HNPCC) 34
    References of polyps 35
Malignant Lymphoma of Gastrointestinal Tract 39
    Extranodal Lymphoma 39
    Malignant Lymphoma of Stomach 40
        Gastric Marginal –Zone B-cell Lymphoma (Extranodal marginal zone B-cell lymphoma of mucosa-associated lymphatic tissue (MALT) type.) 40

Evolution of extranodal marginal zone B-cell lymphoma of mucosa-associated lymphatic tissue (MALT) type and Diffuse Large B Cell Lymphoma 43
    Diffuse large B Cell Lymphoma (DLBCL) of Stomach 43
    Lymphomas of small intestine 44
    Immunoproliferative Small Intestinal Disease (IPSID) 44
    Diffuse Large B cell Lymphoma of Small Intestines 45
    Enteropathy-Type Intestinal T-cell Lymphoma 46
    Mantle Cell Lymphoma & Multiple Lymphomatous Polyposis 47
  References for extranodal lymphoma 50
Gastro-Entero-Pancreatic Endocrine Tumors 53
  The Dispersed Neuroendocrine System 53
  Neuroendocrine tumors of gastrointestinal tract and pancreas 56
    General Considerations (Tables 3.3, 3.4) 56
    Neuroendocrine Tumors (NET) of Stomach 57
    Type 1 gastric carcinoids 58
    Type 2 gastric carcinoids (Zollinger Ellison Syndrome) 59
    Type 3 gastric carcinoids of EC cells 59
    Carcinoid tumors (NETs) of small intestine (including duodenum) 60
    Duodenal Neuroendocrine Tumors 61
    Gastrin-Producing (G cell) neuroendocrine tumors (Gastrinoma) 62
    Somatostatin-Producing (D cell) NET 62
    Serotonin-Producing NET 62
    Gangliocytic Paraganglioma 62
    Jejunal/Ileal Neuroendocrine tumors 64
    Colonic Neuroendocrine Tumor 65
    Recto-sigmoid Neuroendocrine Tumor 65
    Appendicular Neuroendocrine Tumor 65
  Pancreatic Endocrine Tumors (PETs): 68
    Pancreatic Endocrine Tumors 68
    Neurofibromatosis & PETs 70
    Insulinoma, glucagonoma, Gastrinoma and Somatostatinoma will be described and illustrated. 70
    Insulinoma 70
    Glucagonoma 73
    Gastrinoma 75
    Nesidioblastosis 77
  Refrences of Gastro-Entero-Pancreatic Neuroendocrine Tumors 80

PREFACE:

DIAGNOSTIC PROBLEMS IN SURGICAL PATHOLOGY:

Uncommon presentation of common lesions and rare lesions

Histopathological evaluation is the gold standard in the diagnosis of malignant tumors and chronic diseases of visceral organs like liver, kidney and lungs. Histopathological analysis provides information that helps the clinician to choose the most appropriate treatment modality and assists in prognostication. Notwithstanding the current and future advances in the imaging technology and other innovations, the status of Histopathology will remain unchanged for decades to come.

Whereas Histopathology is the most objective form of investigation, there are many gray areas in arriving at a definitive diagnosis. On many occasions total lack of clinical information leads to avoidable errors in the diagnosis. The surgical pathologist is advised to keep the cases pending until adequate information is available. On the other hand there are numerous problems in histological interpretation even if the entire clinical information is at hand. This occurs because some lesions have inherent morphological ambiguities and no two surgical pathologists may agree on the correct histological diagnosis. One such lesion, for example, is verrucous squamous cell carcinoma of the oro-pharyngeal region or other organs with squamous epithelial lining. The most controversial problem in thyroid disorders is a lesion called follicular variant of papillary carcinoma. In every organ and system, there are sporadic entities, which have debatable criteria of morphological diagnosis. The object of this book is to adequately address problems of uncommon morphologic variations of common lesions and rare difficult lesions with the help of extensive illustrations. There are excellent frequently updated textbooks of surgical pathology, in which all lesions occurring in various sites are described, illustrated and backed by references. However, due to constraints of space, these problematic entities are not extensively illustrated or explained at length. This deficiency is admirably handled in exclusively individual organ pathology monograms. However, this requires the facility of a well-stocked library; most practicing surgical pathologists do not have access to these.

The proposed book is an attempt to address these lesions with multiple illustrations and detailed pertinent text. It is envisaged that the book should be a companion to a standard surgical pathology textbook and this should be accessible just at the fingertips via power of electronic media using internet. The targeted audience includes residents in Anatomic Pathology; young recently qualified pathologists and a large contingent of pathologists attached to medical institutions, in which the volume of surgical specimens is low.

Note on statistical data presented in this eBook:

The senior author (ARC) has been a practicing consultant surgical pathologist for the last 44 years (1969-2013). As a surgical pathologist, he has been associated with 'surgical pathology center' (his own lab). He is also attached to the following hospitals in Mumbai (Bombay): Sir H N Hospital, Bombay

Hospital and Jaslok Hospital (all corporate institutions), Bone Registry, Grant Medical College; Cytology department of KEM Hospital.

He has gathered vast amount of neoplastic cases of different organ-systems and the data has been in the form of Tables for different organ systems. The statistical tabulation of tumors has been based on classification of anatomical site and behavior (benign or malignant). This is not purported to be a population based epidemiological data. However, the data likely represents a fair cross sectional distribution and representation of various neoplasms in the population served in Metropolitan Mumbai (Bombay), India.

DISCLAIMER:

This Book titled Diagnostic Problems in Tumors of Gastrointestinal Tract: Selected Topics, is made available by the Authors solely for trained and licensed physician for personal, non-commercial teaching and educational use. No two individual patients with neoplasms are identical and therefore diagnosis and treatment varies greatly depending on the medical and surgical history. The information contained in this Book is not medical advice. It is the professional responsibility of the practitioner to apply the information provided in a specific situation. Attention has been taken for accuracy of the information presented to describe generally accepted practices; however, knowledge and best practice in the field constantly change with new research. Readers are advised to check the most current information. The authors, editors and publishers are not responsible for errors or omissions or for any outcomes from the use of the information in this book and make no warranty, expressed or implied, with respect to the currency, completeness or accuracy of the content of the publication. This educational application is not a medical device and does not and should not be construed to provide health related or medical advice, or clinical decision support or to support or replace the diagnosis, recommendation, advise, treatment or decision by an appropriately trained licensed physician, including, without limitation with respect to any life sustaining or lifesaving treatment or decision. This educational material does not create a physician patient relationship between the authors and any individual. Before making any medical or health related decision, individuals, including those with any neoplasms are advised to consult an appropriately trained and licensed physician. To the fullest extent of the law, the authors, the editors or the publisher do not assume any liability for any injury and/or damage to persons or property arising out of or related to any use of the material contained in this book.

Polyps of Gastrointestinal Tract

Introduction

A polyp is an abnormal growth of tissue projecting from surface of mucous membrane (or skin surface, albeit rarely). It is attached by an elongated stalk, when it is called pedunculated polyp. It is called sessile when it is attached without a stalk.

Polyp is a clinical term or gross description of any circumscribed discrete growth that projects above the surrounding mucosa. The term polyp does not imply any specific disease. The core of the polyp can be hamartomatous, inflammatory or neoplastic [benign or malignant] and a correct diagnosis is arrived at on histological examination of a biopsy or totally resected polyp. Apart from histological examination, significant information of diagnostic significance can be obtained from answers to the following:

I] does the biopsy come from a discrete polyp or a prominent mucosal fold?
II] Is it pedunculated or sessile?
III] Status of surrounding mucosa; is it normal or inflammatory?
IV] Whether polyps are present in other parts of the GI tract?

Thus, clinical, endoscopic gross appearance and histological study are all essential for accurate diagnosis, classification, therapeutic decisions and long-term prognosis of a polyp from any part of the gastrointestinal tract. For an isolated or solitary polyp, which is far more common than syndromic polyposis, concern of its malignant potential is of fundamental importance and type of treatment instituted varies from case to case. Surgical pathologist has a great responsibility in assisting the clinician to make a correct decision for the type of appropriate treatment: mere snaring of the polyp or segmental resection of the bowel bearing the polyp. When the polyp is excised in toto it should be subjected to frozen section analysis. If adenocarcinoma is detected in the head of the polyp and separately sectioned stalk of the polyp is free from malignancy, polypectomy is an adequate treatment. If the stalk is involved segmental bowel resection is required.

A large variety of polyposis syndromes, hereditary or non-hereditary, occur in the gastrointestinal system. An accurate classification of a polyp often gives a clue to possibility of a polyposis syndrome. Patients of syndromic polyposis require special forms of treatment including long term surveillance and surgical intervention during the life of these cases.

In this section, only selected types of polyps, particularly those with epithelial proliferation and those with dysplasia or progression to cancer will be described. It can not be too strongly emphasized that classification of polyps is not easy when small biopsies are available for evaluation, for there is a considerable overlap in different types of polyps, particularly in stomach. Mesenchymal tumors like gist, leiomyoma or leiomyosarcoma, lipoma etc do present as polypoid masses and these lesions will be briefly referred to.

Polyps of Stomach

Benign gastric polyps are reported in 3%-5% of patients undergoing EGD endoscopy and the most common polyps have been hyperplastic or inflammatory and fundic gland types (60% and 30% respectively), followed by adenomas (10-15%). These Figureures are derived from studies conducted over long periods of time in relatively small numbers of patients.(1) There are hardly any reports on gastric polyps in the Indian literature and the prevalence of various types of polyps is not known. The Author has mainly seen hyperplastic polyps and few fundic gland polyps. Adenomatous polyp is indeed rare in our experience. Carmack et al (1) presented the data on current spectrum of gastric polyps in a 1-year National Study of over 120,000 patients. The most common indications for endoscopy included GERD (38.6%), dyspepsia or epigastric pain (18%) and anemia (8.3%). The cases were accrued from private practices of 36 states in the US. The results are as follows: prevalence of gastric polyps in the EGD population was 6.35%; 77% were fundic gland polyps, 17% hyperplastic polyps/polypoid foveolar hyperplasia, 0.69% adenomatous polyps, and 0.1% inflammatory fibroid polyps. The study is huge and Figureures statistically valid.

Hyperplastic Polyp:

Synonyms: inflammatory, regenerative or hyperplasiogenous polyp

Definition

The hyperplastic gastric polyp is usually about 5 mm in size and characterized by foveolar proliferation, scattered cystic glands and inflammatory lamina propria. They account for 75-90% of all gastric polyps and in vast majority of cases occur in a background of long standing chronic gastritis (2, 3).

Clinical Findings

These polyps are found most often in older patients and occur equally in both sexes. About 50% are about 5 mm in size and many others are between 5 and 10 mm. In a series of 160 hyperplastic polyps (3), 137 [85%] polyps were accompanied by background chronic gastritis. H pylori gastritis [25%], chemical gastropathy [21.6%] and autoimmune gastritis [12%] were encountered in this study. It has been suggested that hyperplastic polyp develops as a consequence of exaggerated mucosal response to tissue injury and inflammation. In fact, regression of hyperplastic polyps has been documented in 71% of patients with H Pylori infection after irradication of bacterial infection (4). In the opinion of this author inflammatory polyp is perhaps a more appropriate term than hyperplastic polyp.

Microscopic

Microscopic examination reveals marked foveolar proliferation with elongated distorted and branched foveolae, scattered cystic glands and excess edematous vascular lamina propria with diffuse infiltrate of lymphocytes, plasma cells and few neutrophils (Figure 1.1). Dysplasia is a rare finding in hyperplastic polyps and case reports of carcinoma occurring in hyperplastic polyps do appear in the literature. It is accepted that hyperplastic polyp has no significant precancerous role but the background chronic gastritis is conducive to induce neoplastic changes. However, it is recommended that larger polyps of the size above 1.5 cm should be completely resected endoscopically. It has been observed that gastric mucosa surrounding the polyps may reveal dysplasia or adenocarcinoma, which are exceptionally seen to arise in the polyps. Hence, the gastroenterologist must take gastric mucosal biopsies surrounding the polyp to assess the presence of dysplastic changes and rarely carcinoma.

There are many types of gastric polyps with certain common histological features and differentiation cannot be readily achieved without proper study and clinico-pathological correlation. Polypoid foveolar hyperplasia, gastric foveolar polyp and gastritis cystica profunda are difficult to differentiate from hyperplastic polyp but they have also been described as morphological variants of hyperplastic polyp. Polyp associated with Menetrier's disease, polyp of Cronkhite Canada syndrome and juvenile polyps are almost indistinguishable from hyperplastic polyps.

The definition of hyperplastic gastric polyp is still evolving. In a recent paper on a review of 208 polyps initially diagnosed as HP, 41 cases (20%) were considered typical HP, 103 cases (49%) were classified as polypoid foveolar hyperplasia and 64 cases (31%) diagnosed as mucosal prolapse polyps. The latter is located in antrum, which has pronounced peristalsis. This leads to mucosal prolapse and development of the polyp. (5)

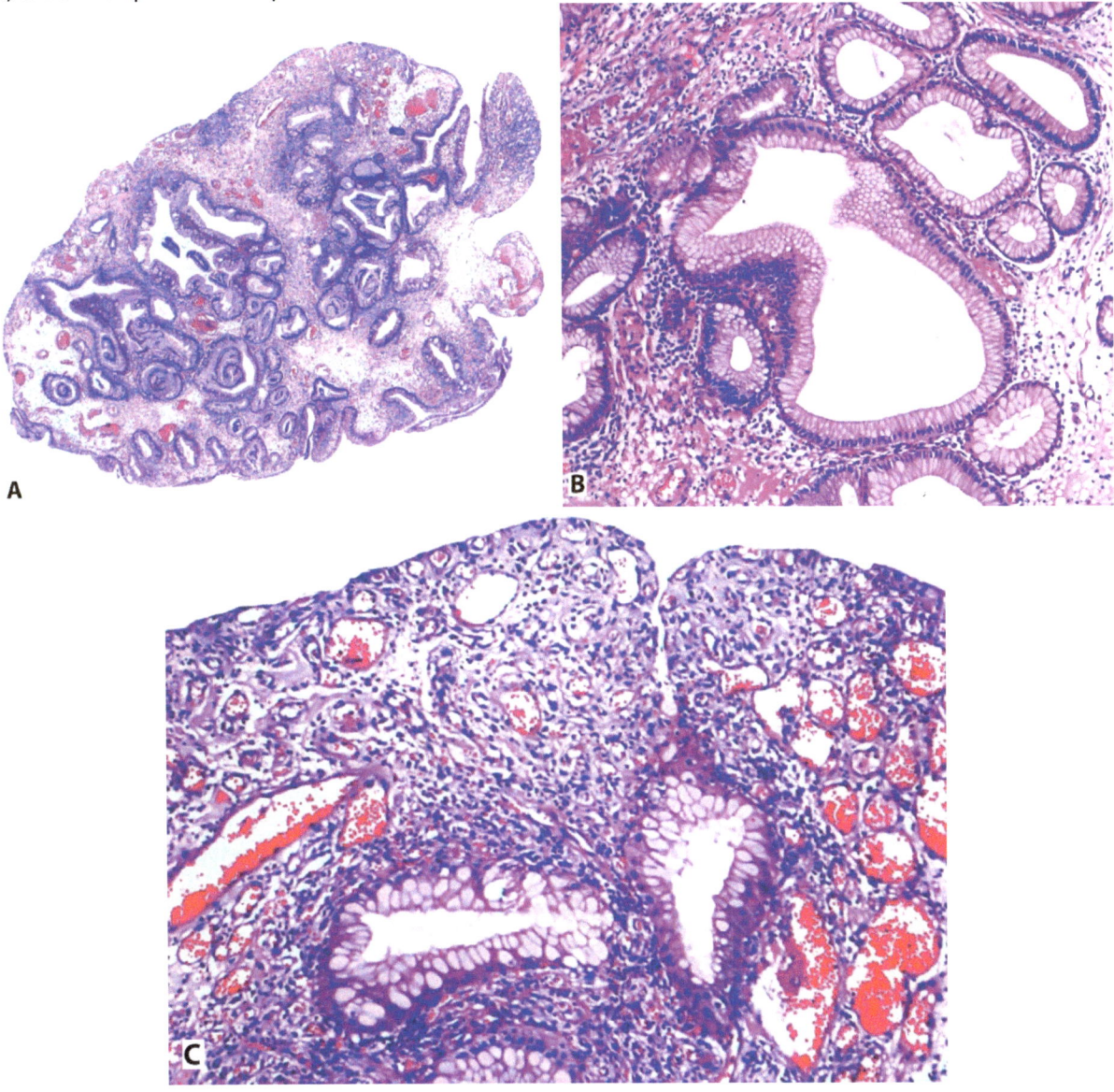

Figure 1.1 Hyperplastic gastric polyp: (A) scanner view of polyp showing ulceration, inflammation and dilated or cystic glands (B) dilated foveolar glands and inflammatory lamina propria (C) ulcerated surface epithelium, intense inflammation, glandular destruction, and excess engorged vessels

Fundic Gland Polyp (FGP):

Definition:

Fundic gland polyps are common and occur in gastric body and fundus. They are typically small (1-5 mm) and composed of dilated or cystic glands lined by mixture of attenuated parietal cells, chief cells and mucous neck cells.

Clinical Findings

FGPs are sporadic or associated with hereditary diseases like familial adenomatous polyposis (FAP), attenuated FAP syndromes, Peutz-Jeghers syndrome and juvenile polyposis (6,7). They have been reported in non-hereditary disorders like Zollinger-Ellison syndrome and atrophic gastritis. The incidence of fundic polyp has dramatically increased because of their association with proton pump inhibitor therapy (8, 9). The latter is particularly responsible for frequent occurrence of fundic gland polyposis. Whereas, hyperplastic polyp often develops in H Pylori infected gastric mucosa; prevalence of H pylori infection is rather low in fundic polyps.

Recent studies have suggested that fundic gland polyps in FAP are truly neoplastic, showing mutation of APC gene. These FGPs are truly neoplastic, have 25 to 50% prevalence of dysplasia and may rarely give rise to adenocarcinoma. In contrast, sporadic fundic polyps and those associated with proton inhibitor drugs show no dysplasia or APC gene mutation.

Microscopic

It is usually easy to differentiate this polyp from hyperplastic polyp, although both typically show cystic glands. The glands in fundic polyp are lined by parietal and chief cells those of hyperplastic polyp only by foveolar epithelium. A few foveolar glands are also seen in the former but unlike the hyperplastic polyp the lamina propria is uninflamed (Figure 1.2).

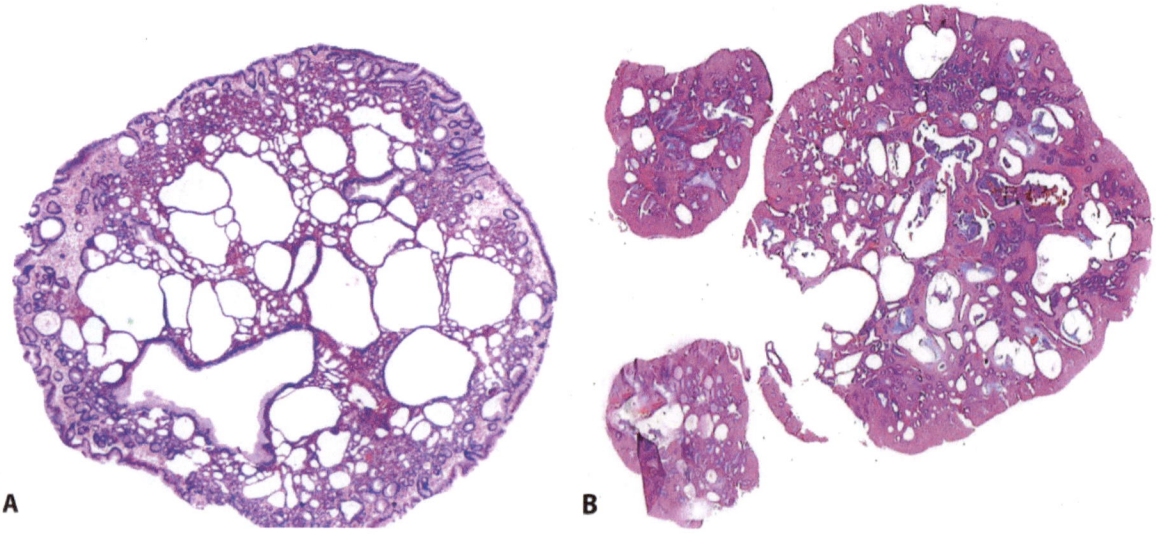

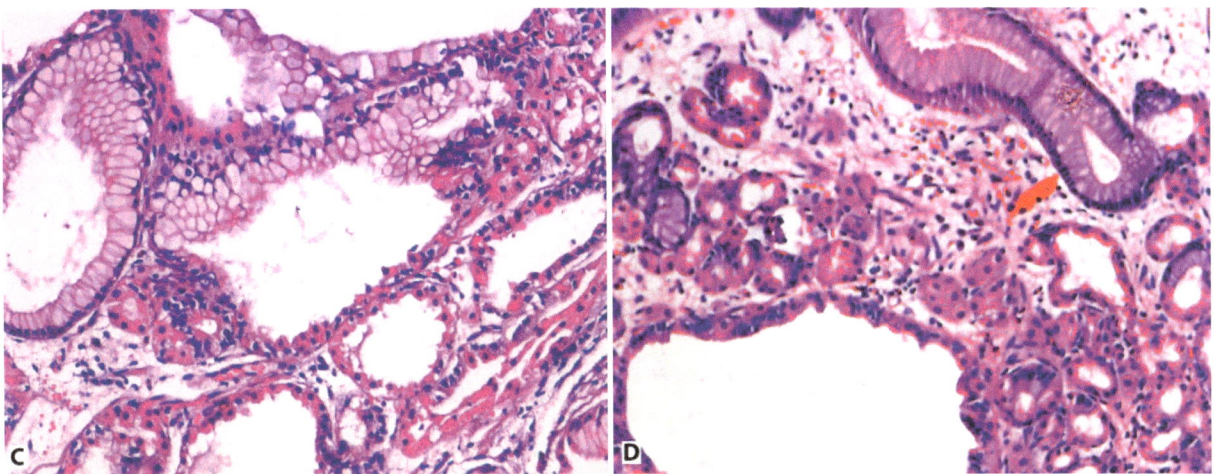

Figure 1.2 Fundic gland polyposis: (A & B) scanner view of multiple fundic polyps (C & D) cystic glands lined by normal parietal and few foveolar cells; no inflammation in lamina propria

Adenomatous Polyp (Gastric adenoma):

Definition

Adenomatous polyp is a neoplastic growth characterized by localized polypoid proliferation of dysplastic epithelium and frequently occurs in stomach with a background of mucosal atrophy and intestinal metaplasia. In most publications it accounts for 7-10% of all gastric polyps (1).

Clinical findings

Gastric adenoma occurs as a solitary sessile or pedunculated polyp, usually less than 2 cm, [large 3-4 cm] (Figure 1.3 A, B) and which is asymptomatic until it bleeds, ulcerates or causes gastric outflow obstruction. Gastric adenomas are associated with a high risk of malignancy, the risk related to the size of the lesion. It is particularly high in lesions that are greater than 2 cm (10). In view of their established precancerous role in the genesis of gastric adenocarcinoma, the polyps must be removed in toto and surrounding gastric mucosa sampled to look for inflammation and intestinal metaplasia (11).

Microscopic

The adenomatous polyp closely resembles colorectal adenoma and shows the same range of dysplastic changes and architecturally divisible into tubular, tubulovillous and villous. Gastric adenomatous polyps are classified as intestinal type when these are composed of intestinal type columnar epithelium with goblet cells. Paneth cells, endocrine differentiation and even brush border are present. The gastric adenoma (foveolar type) is lined entirely by dysplastic gastric mucin cells containing a neutral mucin on PAS-alcian blue stain. Majority of such adenomas occurred in association with familial adenomatous polyposis (FAP)

In a study of 61 gastric adenomas (12) 82% were solitary and contained adenocarcinoma in nine cases (14.8%) (Figure 1.3). There were 34 (56%) intestinal type adenomas and 25 (41%) gastric adenomas. The intestinal type adenomas are more likely to show high grade dysplasia, adenocarcinoma in polyp and intestinal metaplasia in the surrounding stomach, than gastric type adenoma. The frequency of adenocarcinoma developing from dysplasia of gastric adenoma seems to vary considerably. In one study, long term follow up of gastric adenomas with low grade dysplasia showed no progression to cancer and in one case of high grade dysplasia the lesion progressed to intra mucosal carcinoma with no instance of invasion into submucosa or beyond (13).

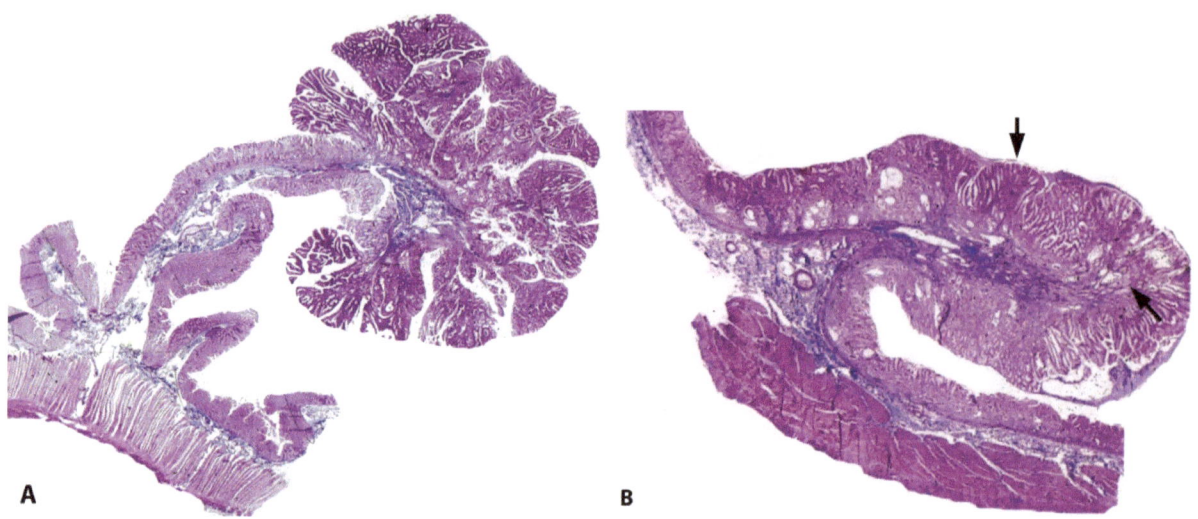

Figure 1.3 Whole mount section of adenomatous polyps of stomach: (A) adenocarcinoma in situ in the head of the polyp, note lack of infiltration in the stalk of the polyp (B) adenomatous polyp with intramucosal adenocarcinoma (arrows) but no invasion

Polyps of Small Intestines

Brunner Gland Adenoma:

Synonyms: Brunneroma, Brunner gland hyperplasia.

The last word has not been said about the nature of this entity and precise definition is not possible. Most investigators tend to believe that the lesion is non-neoplastic and therefore not an adenoma or adenomatous polyp. Brunner glands extend from the distal pylorus to a variable distance, stopping at the first or second part of the duodenum. The glands secrete alkaline fluid composed of viscous mucin, which protects duodenal epithelium from the acid chime of the stomach.

Clinical Findings

The lesion is often detected incidentally during endoscopy or may be large enough to elicit signs of obstruction or hemorrhage. Two cases of duodenal intussusception associated with Brunner gland lesion, one with a fatal hemorrhage, have been reported (14). In a study of 120 patients with chronic renal failure multinodular filling defects were seen in duodenal wall in 28 cases, associated with severe degree of uremia (15).

Microscopic:

Brunner gland adenoma (Figure 1.4 A, B) consists of nodular hyperplasia of normal Brunner glands (Figure 1.4 C-D) but some comprise mixture of Bruner's glands, cystic ducts, adipose tissue and lymphoid tissue. In a case reported as Brunner gland hamartoma, a 3.5 cm polyp was excised with part of duodenum and it revealed a large adipose component, lobules of hyperplastic Brunner's glands and cystic duct glands lined by ciliated cells (16). In view of these histological findings, Brunner gland hamartoma will be a more appropriate designation. About 150 cases of this lesion have been reported in the literature.

The reported cases have not shown unequivocal de novo neoplasia within Brunner glands, although secondary involvement of Brunner's glands by dysplasia or carcinoma arising in the surface epithelium has been described. Hence some authorities prefer the term Brunner gland hamartoma rather than adenoma, emphasizing an essentially non-neoplastic nature of this lesion (17, 18).

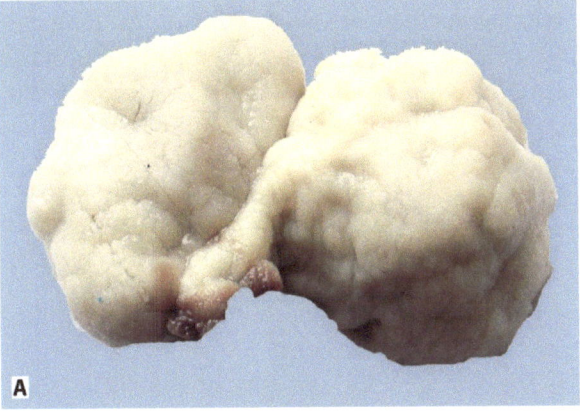 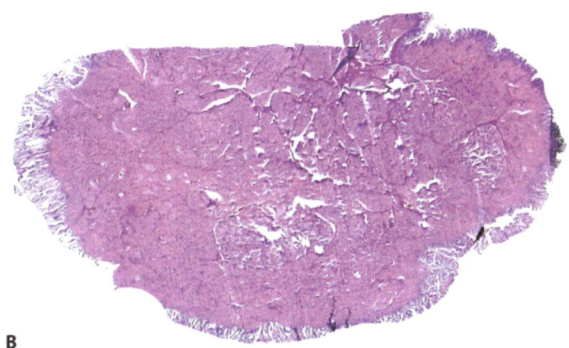

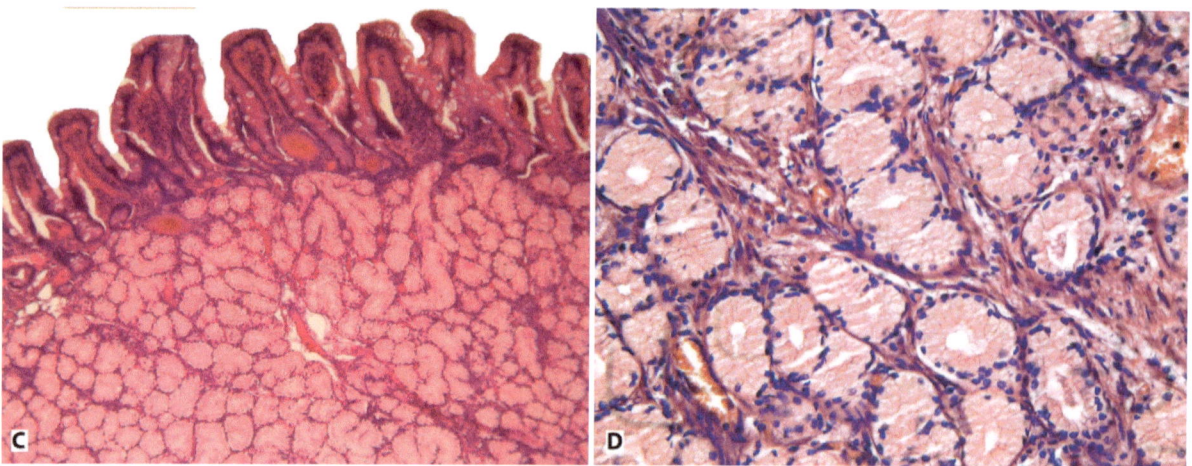

Figure 1.4 Bruner gland adenoma/polyp: (A) bilobed 2.5 cm polyp, (B) whole mount section of Brunner gland polyp, (C) low power view of the polyp, (D) high power of constituent Brunner's glands

Inflammatory Fibroid Polyp:

Synonyms: Eosinophilic granuloma, inflammatory pseudotumor, fibroma, hemangiopericytoma etc

Definition

Inflammatory fibroid polyp is a rare mesenchymal tumor of the gastrointestinal tract that consists of spindle shaped stromal cells and an infiltrate rich in eosinophils.

This is uncommon benign non-neoplastic inflammatory polyp occurring throughout the gastrointestinal tract with predilection to small intestine and stomach, and less commonly large intestine. It is composed of edematous vascular fibrous tissue with a variety of inflammatory cells dominated by eosinophils.

Most observers consider inflammatory fibroid polyp to be a form of reactive pseudotumor. Although the histogenesis of this polyp remains controversial, a possible origin from dendritic cells or CD-34 positive perivascular cells has been proposed

Clinical Findings

The polyps are usually solitary, 2 to 5 cm in size, initially sessile and over a period of time become pedunculated and ulcerated (Figure 1.5 A). The small sized lesions are discovered incidentally at endoscopy and large lesions may cause obstructive symptoms such as nausea vomiting and abdominal pain. In some cases the polyp can cause intussusception. Initially IFP was thought to be part of the spectrum of eosinophilic gastroenteritis because of significant tissue eosinophilia in the polyp. However, no consistent relationship with atopic, alimentary allergies, parasitic infection or peripheral eosinophilia has been demonstrated (19).

Microscopic:

The lesion is mainly submucosal and composed of vascular fibroblastic proliferation with diffuse infiltrate of lymphocytes, plasma cells, histiocytes and large population of eosinophils (Figure 1.5 B, C). The spindle cells within the lesion are typically arranged around arterioles. The histogenesis and role of spindly stromal cells have been the subjects of extensive immunohistochemical study. These cells express vimentin, CD34, Bcl2 and smooth muscle actin and are negative for S-100, , CD 117 and desmin. The results of this study confirm the presence of myofibroblastic and histiocytic lines of differentiation in addition to the fibroblastic features of the main cellular component in IFP (20).

The earlier reports on immunohistochemical studies showed reactivity to CD34 and C-kit and suggested that IFP may be related to GIST. However, the recent study led to the conclusion that stromal cells in IFP are of dendritic cell origin with possible myofibroblastic differentiation and that they are unrelated to GIST (21).

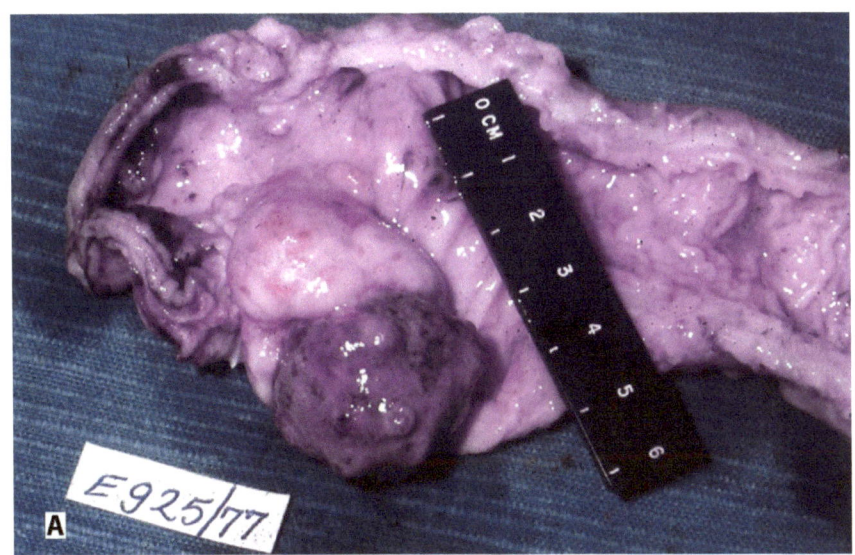

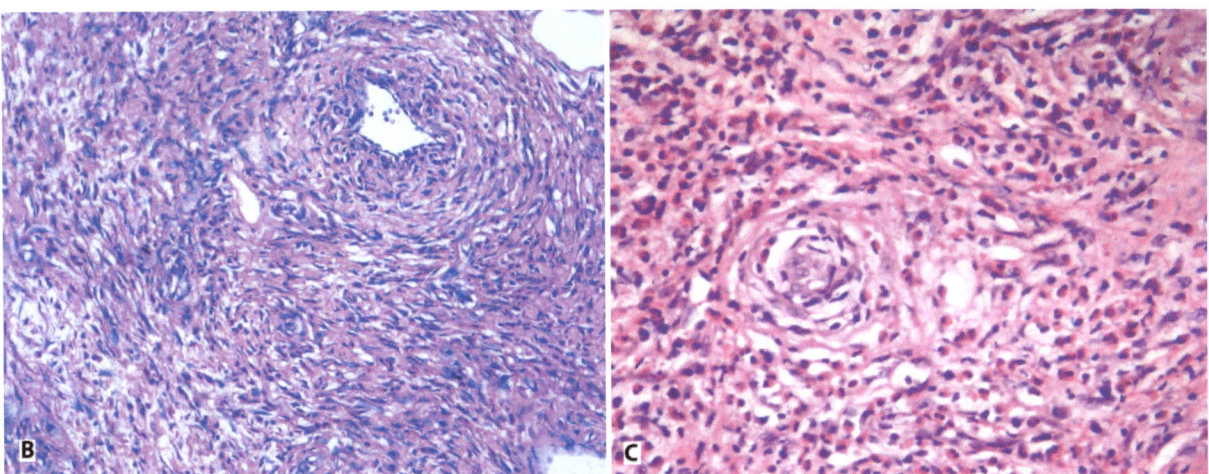

Figure 1.5 Inflammatory fibroid polyp: (A) a 4 x 3 cm pedunculated whitish polyp producing dilatation and partial obstruction of small intestine; (B & C) whirling fibroblastic stroma permeated by lymphoplasmacytic cells and a very rich eosinophilic infiltrate The lesion used to be called localized eosinophilic enteritis.

Colorectal Polyps

(Table 1.1 A) LESIONS OF LARGE BOWEL n=8900 Author's series [1970-2009]	
Inflammatory [non-specific]	1335 [15.6%]
Inflammatory [specific]	148 [1.73%]
Crohn's disease	096 [1.13%]
Ulcerative colitis	2138 [25.0%]
Tuberculosis	596 [6.98%]
Polyps	890 [10.4%]
Benign	265 [3.10%]
Malignant	3067 [35.9%]
Inflammatory [non-spe]	1335 [15.6%]
Inflammatory [specific]	148 [1.73%]

(Table 1.1 B) POLYPS OF LARGE BOWEL n= 923 Author's series [1970-2009]	
Adenomatous	482 [52.2%]
Polyposis	008 [0.87%]
Villous adenoma	067 [7.26%]
Inflammatory	075 [8.13%]
Juvenile	273 [29.6%]
Adenoma malignum	018 [1.77%]

Adenomatous Polyp

Synonyms: Adenoma, tubular adenoma (Tables 1.1, 1.2, 1.3, 1.4, 1.5)

Definition

An adenomatous polyp, sessile or pedunculated (Figure 1.6 A), is defined as neoplastic proliferation of colonic epithelium giving rise to tubular glands with nuclear stratification, mitotic activity and decreased goblet cells. Presence of dysplasia of some degree and variable component of villous differentiation are present. The polyp is subdivided into tubular adenoma, tubulovillous adenoma and villous adenoma. The tumor is of great clinical importance because of its established premalignant role in the genesis of colorectal carcinoma.

Clinical findings

Majority of patients are asymptomatic and some present with occult or overt bleeding. The large polyps may lead to iron deficiency anemia. There is a high prevalence of adenomatous polyps at autopsy, to the tune of 60% in the Western world (high incidence of colorectal cancer) and only 5% in the underdeveloped countries (relatively low incidence of colorectal cancer). By fifth decade of life about 12% of individuals harbor adenomas and approximately 25% of these are high grade lesions (22). The development of adenomas in some individuals is strongly influence by family history (23, 24, 25). This issue will be further discussed in the text on hereditary non-polyposis colorectal cancer.

Microscopic

Adenomatous polyps are sessile or pedunculated (Figure 6A) and consist of thick hyperplastic enlarged mucosal glands arranged compactly (Figure 1.6 B-C) and may exhibit mild, moderate or severe dysplasia. Currently severe dysplasia is considered synonymous with the term carcinoma in situ. Size of the polyp is of great predictive value and polyps less than 1 cm rarely progress to adenocarcinoma. Larger polyps (>2 cm) show severe dysplasia (Figure 1.7 A, B, C) and the atypical glandular proliferation may extend up to muscularis mucosae. Infiltration in the stalk of the polyp beyond muscularis mucosae constitutes an invasive adenocarcinoma (Figureure 1.8A, B, C). There is a 10% to 20% risk of carcinoma at the time of the removal of a large polyp (2 cm size-Figure 1.7 A), whereas, adenoma measuring between 1 and 2 cm has a 5% risk of harboring cancer (26, 27) The amount of villous component in an adenomatous polyp is an important predictive factor in the development of adenocarcinoma (Figure 1.9 A). As a matter of convention, tubular adenomas are estimated to contain 0% to 25% villous component, tubulovillous adenoma 26% to 75% and villous adenoma 76% to100%. The degree of villous differentiation has been shown to increase with increasing size of the adenoma (Figure 1.9 B, C) (28, 29).

The incidence of different types of adenomatous polyps in one very large series of 5786 cases (30) was: 64.5% tubular, 26.6% tubulovillous and 8.9% villous. This series revealed an experience of 1831 patients with adenoma, of which 361 cases revealed carcinoma in situ (20%) and 182 cases of invasive carcinoma (10%). In a series of 3002 patients with colorectal adenoma 19.7% had benign or malignant synchronous tumors and 6% metachronous tumors (31). A large villo-glandular polyp with invasive carcinoma in the core is illustrated in Figure 1.8.

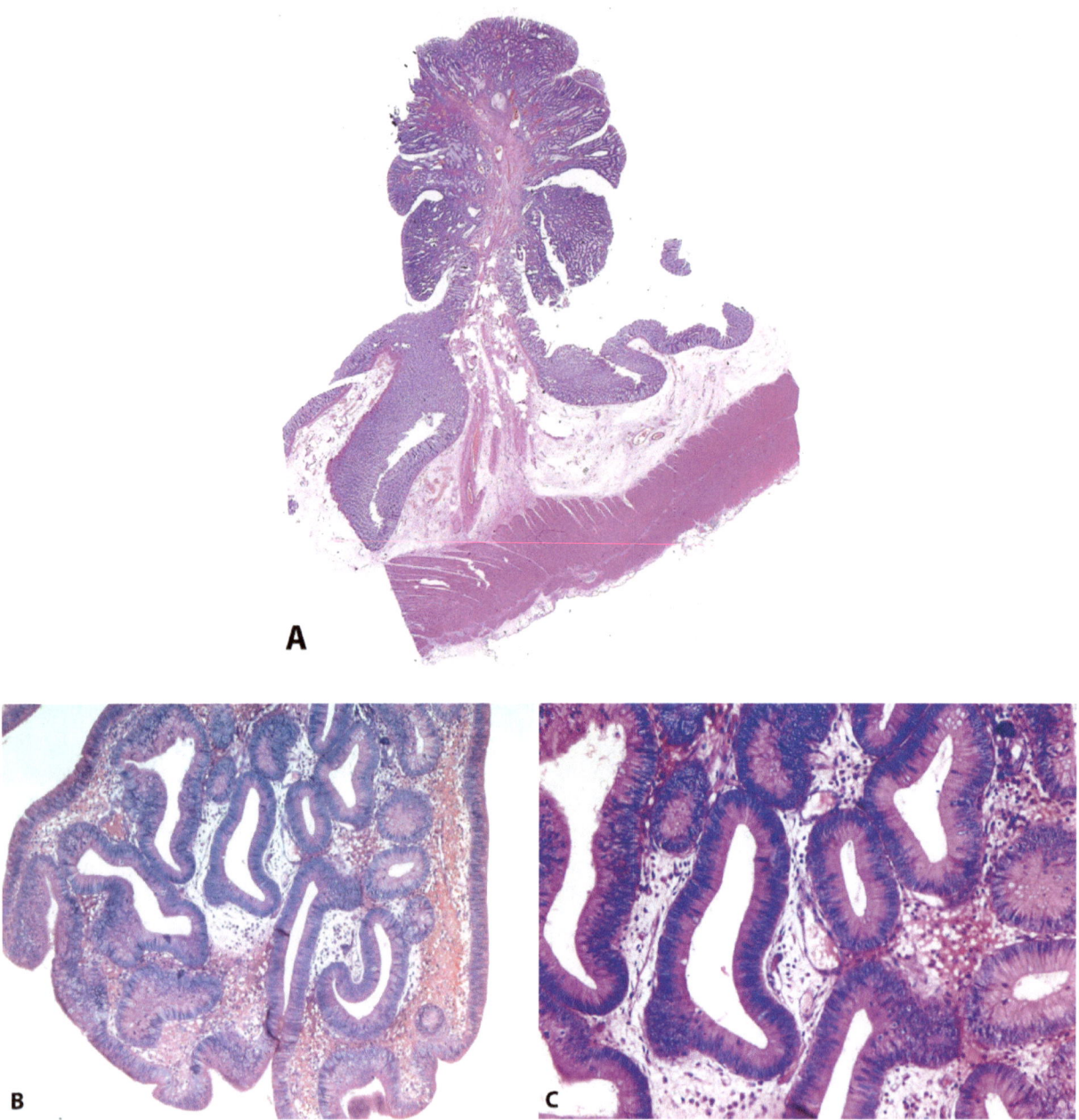

Figure 1.6 Adenomatous polyp: (A) A pedunculated adenomatous polyp of sigmoid incidentally found at autopsy in a case of cardiac tamponade, (B & C) thick mildly hyperchromatic crowded glands almost devoid of mucin,

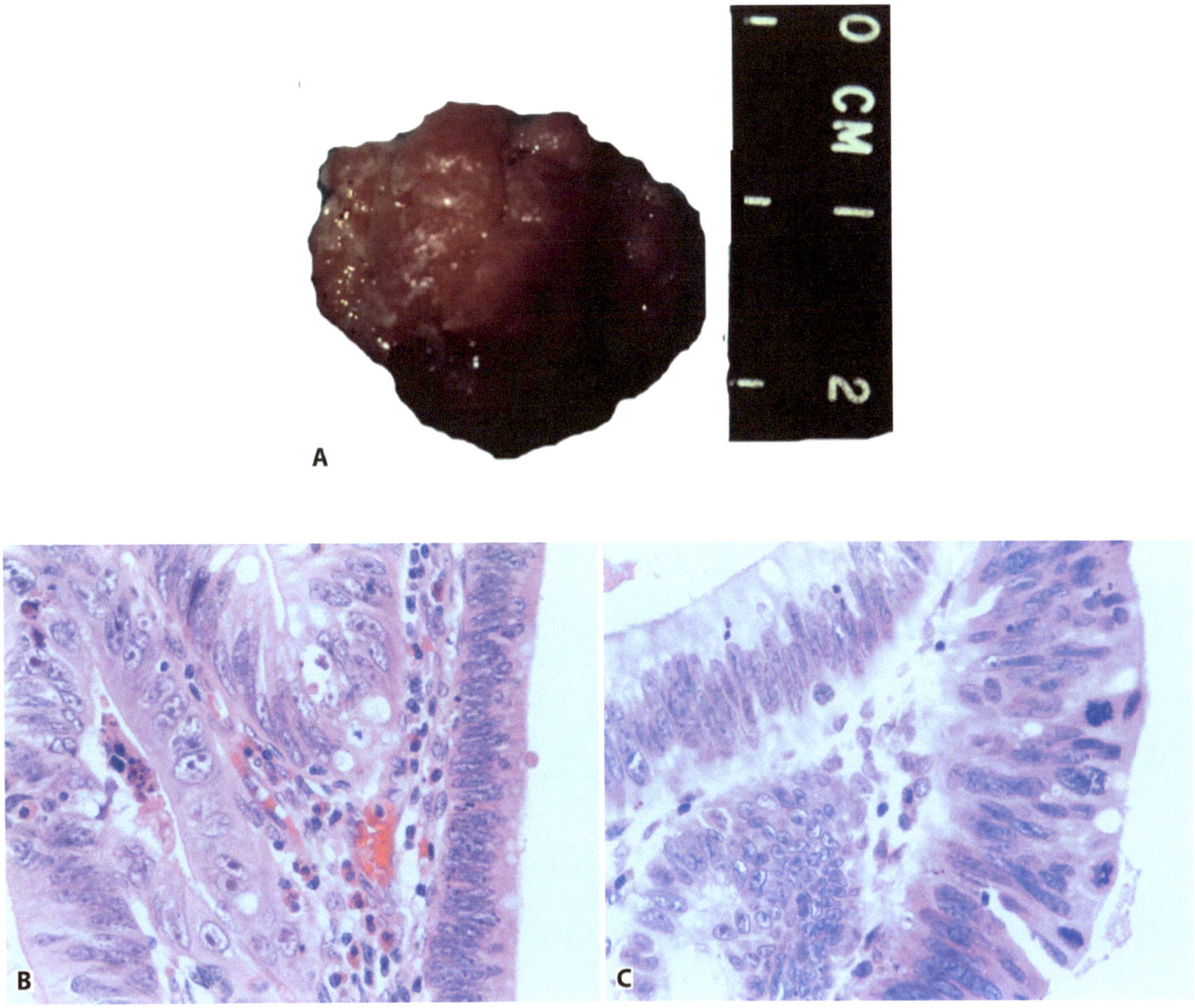

Figure 1.7 (A) a 2 cm sessile colonic polyp (B & C) severe dysplasia (CIS) in superficial glands of the polyp but no stromal invasion in the stalk was found

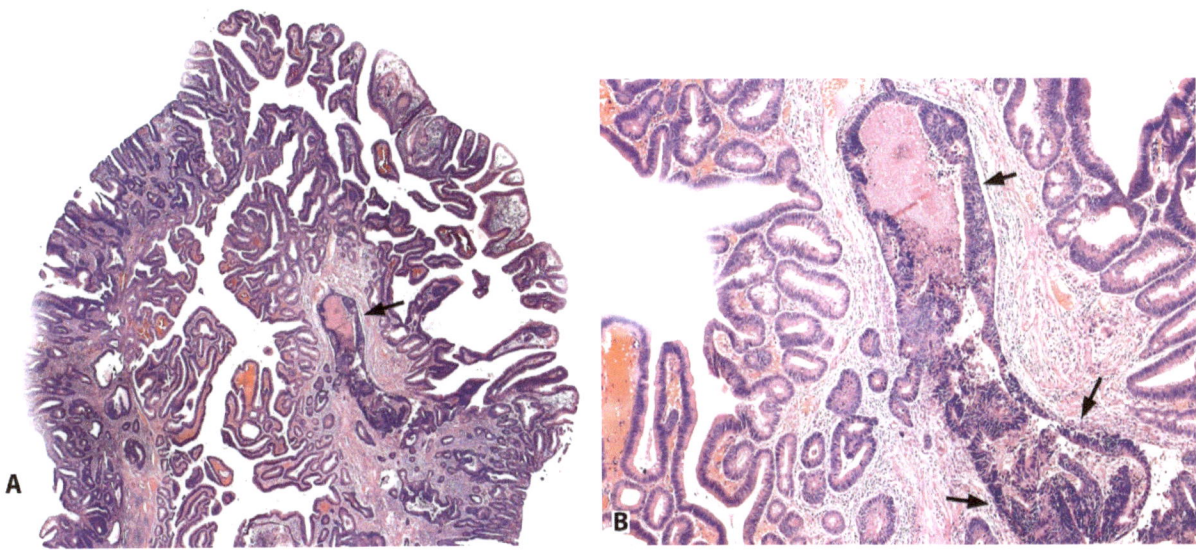

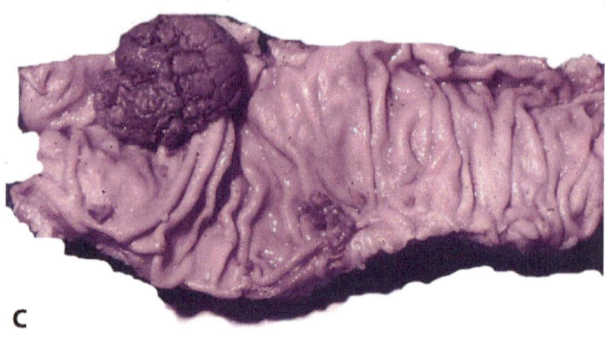

Figure 1.8 (A) Tubulovillous adenoma with high grade dysplasia & architectural complexity (B) invasive adenocarcinoma with desmoplasia in the stalk (arrows). (C) Sigmoid colon was resected following the report above, a single focus of residual adenocarcinoma was found in the submucosa

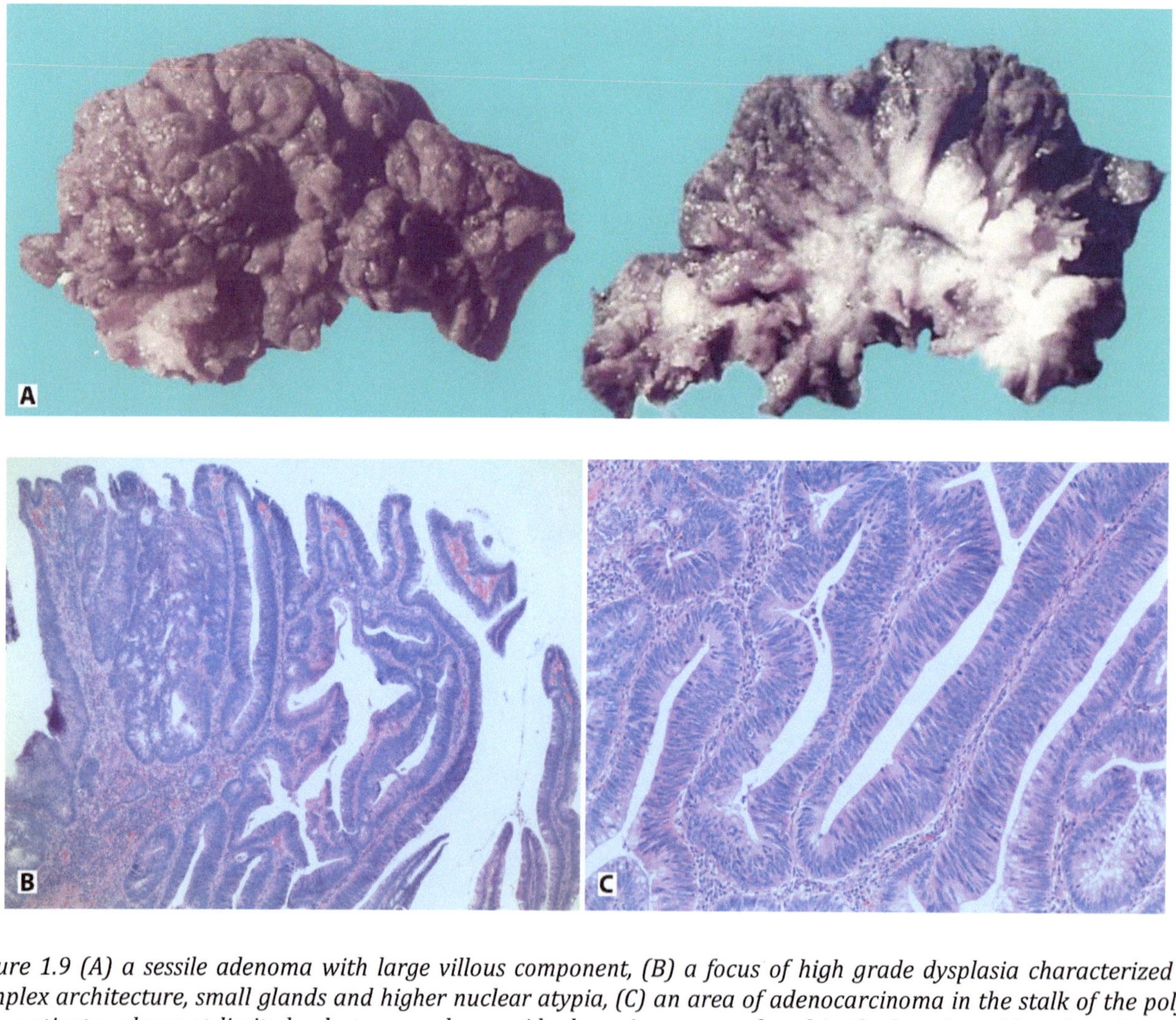

Figure 1.9 (A) a sessile adenoma with large villous component, (B) a focus of high grade dysplasia characterized by complex architecture, small glands and higher nuclear atypia, (C) an area of adenocarcinoma in the stalk of the polyp. This patient underwent limited colectomy and no residual carcinoma was found in the bowel, and lymph nodes were clear. In this case (carcinoma remained confined to the polyp stalk and did not progress to submucosa.

The classification of adenomatous polyps, and malignant potential according to the size and proportion of villous component are presented in Table 1.2. Our experience of prevalence of Crohn's disease, ulcerative colitis, number of adenomatous polyps and adenocarcinoma of right colon is compared with that of left colon is given in Table 1.3.

The malignant potential is directly proportional to the size of the polyp, those with size $\geq$ 2 cm reveal malignant transformation in about 45% of the cases. The malignant potential is also dependent on histological features with particular reference to proportion of tubular and villous components. Adenomatous polyp containing $\geq$75% will have about 45% chance of malignant change.

Table 1.2 Classification of Adenomatous Polyps:	
Tubular	
Villous A (1%-25% villous)	*Tubular*
Villous B (26%-75% villous)	*Tubulovillous*
Villous C (76%-99% villous)	*Villous*
Villous D (100% villous)	
Dysplasia (mild)	Tubular adenoma
Dysplasia (moderate)	High grade dysplasia Carcinoma in situ
Dysplasia (severe)	
(Terms in italics represent WHO classification)	

Table 1.3 Right Colon (total 707 cases) Versus Left Colon (total 5457 cases) Author's series (1970-2009)				
	Crohn's	UC	Polyps	Malignant
Right	57 (8%)	46 (6.5%)	49 (6.9%)	555 (78.5%)
Left	37 (0.7%)	2092 (38.3)	831 (15.2%)	2497 (45.8%)

Serrated Polyps

1) Hyperplastic polyp
2) Sessile Serrated Polyp.
3) Sessile Serrated Adenoma
4) Mixed Hyperplastic and adenomatous Polyp

This is a heterogeneous group of polypoid lesions of large bowel morphologically characterized by serrated [saw toothed or stellate] architecture of the epithelial component. There is a significant confusion on the precise histological definition and classification. The term hyperplastic polyp without a modifier is acceptable. Sessile serrated polyp and sessile serrated adenoma are currently considered as synonymous and acceptable terms {WHO, 2010}.

Hyperplastic Polyp (HP)

Definition

Hyperplastic polyp is a serrated polyp, rather small (1 to 5 mm) and innocuous, occurring throughout the colon but particularly in rectum. It reveals serrated surface due to papillary infoldings of vacuolated mucinous surface epithelium, and star shaped glands beneath.

Clinical Findings

Usually an incidental finding, its prevalence increasing with age and vast majority occur in left colon (32). Factors associated with hyperplastic polyps include smoking, alcohol consumption, low residue diet and obesity (33). Endoscopically, the polyps are small sessile, button like nodules that appear pale. It is usually left alone but biopsy may be carried out if it can not be distinguished from adenoma on endoscopy.

Microscopic

Hyperplastic polyps are non-dysplastic serrated polyps and sub-classified into three types: microvesicular, goblet cell and mucin poor (34). However, these are mere morphological variations and of no clinical relevance. The glands in the core of the polyp are typically star shaped (Figure 1.10 A & B).

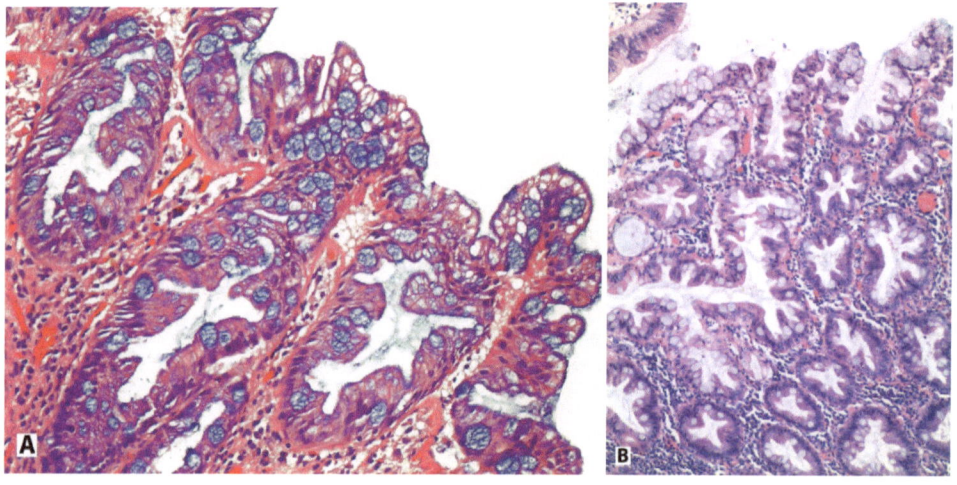

Figure 1.10 Hyperplastic polyp: (A) superficial serrations and elongated superficial star shaped glands containing mucinous cells (B) lower part of polyp has dilated serrated star shaped crypts

Are Hyperplastic polyps related to the genesis of colorectal cancer?

HP was first described in 1926 and distinguished from villous papilloma and solid adenoma. All these decades it has been considered to be a non-neoplastic lesion with no malignant potential (35). In an earlier study of 171 cases of HP, 13% showed foci of adenomatous change (35). There is now strong evidence to suggest that the hyperplastic polyp is not harmless but apparently serves as the precursor of colorectal cancer with DNA methylation and deficient DNA mismatch repair (36). This novel pathway, now called as serrated pathway, applies particularly to the subset of hyperplastic polyps that occur in the proximal colon. This form of hyperplastic polyp is called sessile serrated polyp (further described below). Chung et al proposed that the term "sessile serrated polyp" should be restricted to large (>1 cm) proximally located polyps with a presumed biologic risk (37).

Sessile Serrated Polyp (SSP) Without Dysplasia

Synonyms: Atypical hyperplastic polyp, hyperplastic polyp with architectural abnormalities, large hyperplastic polyp, etc.

Definition

This is a type of hyperplastic polyp, which is characterized by size larger than 0.5 to 1cm, sessile growth pattern, architectural abnormalities and its occurrence in right colon.

Clinical Findings

It may be incidentally detected during colonoscopy or may be found in vicinity of an adenocarcinoma in the right colon. Large sized SSP are often symptomatic and may harbor adenocarcinoma in situ or early invasive adenocarcinoma.

Microscopic

SSP is characterized by crypt dilatation, irregular branched and horizontal crypts, prominent lower crypt serrations, mitoses in upper levels of the crypts, vesicular nuclei in upper crypts, reduced amount of lamina propria between crypts and hypermucinous epithelium (Figure 1.11) (34, 39). There is no significant histological difference between SSP and SSA except that SSA is composed of cells with abundant acidophilic cytoplasm and show variable dysplasia. The reader is advised to use the term SSA, interchangeable with SSP. It is evident that sessile serrated lesions form a histological continuum from hyperplastic polyp to SSP and SSA.

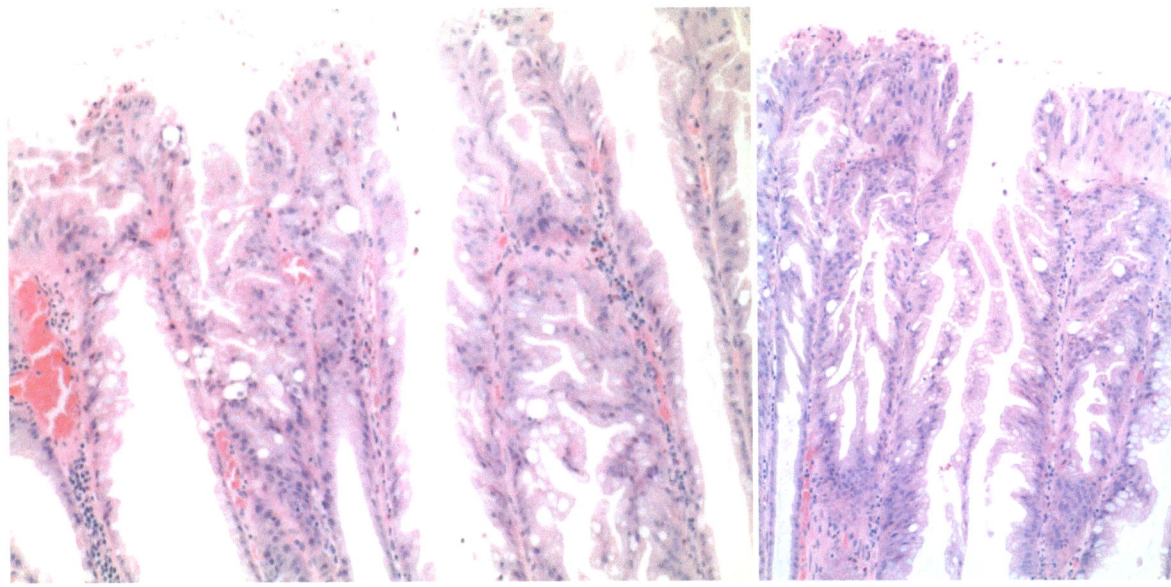

Figure 1.11 Sessile serrated polyp: villiform upper parts of crypts, serrations all the way to deeper part of the crypts and hypermucinous glandular epithelium. Histology almost similar to that of sessile serrated adenoma (see Figure 12)

Sessile Serrated Adenoma

Definition

It is characterized by epithelium with confluent pink eosinophilic cytoplasm and a papillary or villiform growth pattern.

In one series of 110 cases of mixed hyperplastic and adenomatous polyps 37% contained foci of significant dysplasia and 11% contained areas of intramucosal carcinoma. The authors (38) concluded that these lesions reflect a morphologically unique variant of adenoma and suggested that they be termed "serrated adenoma" (also termed sessile serrated adenoma) in order to emphasize their neoplastic nature.

Clinical Findings

These are common in females and endoscopically the polyp appears pedunculated; in one study 63% were pedunculated, 29% sessile and 8% flat or carpet like (32, 43).

Microscopic

Histigically, the adenomas are characterized by prominent crypt serration with confluent epithelial dysplasia, depleted mucin, micropapillation of the surface epithelium and cells with eosinophilic cytoplasm (Figure 1.12 A, B, C) (39, 42, 44).

Serrated adenoma shows dysplastic changes, namely: marked nuclear atypia and nuclear stratification at all levels. A large polyp may reveal areas of conventional adenoma and this type of lesion has been referred to as mixed conventional/serrated adenoma. (9) In one study, progression to dysplasia was reported in 37% of serrated adenomas (38).

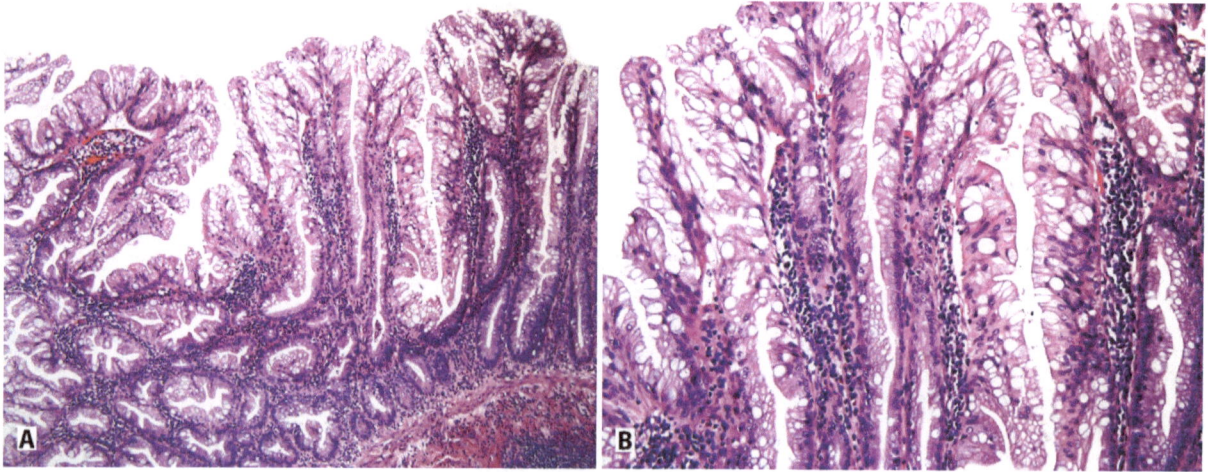

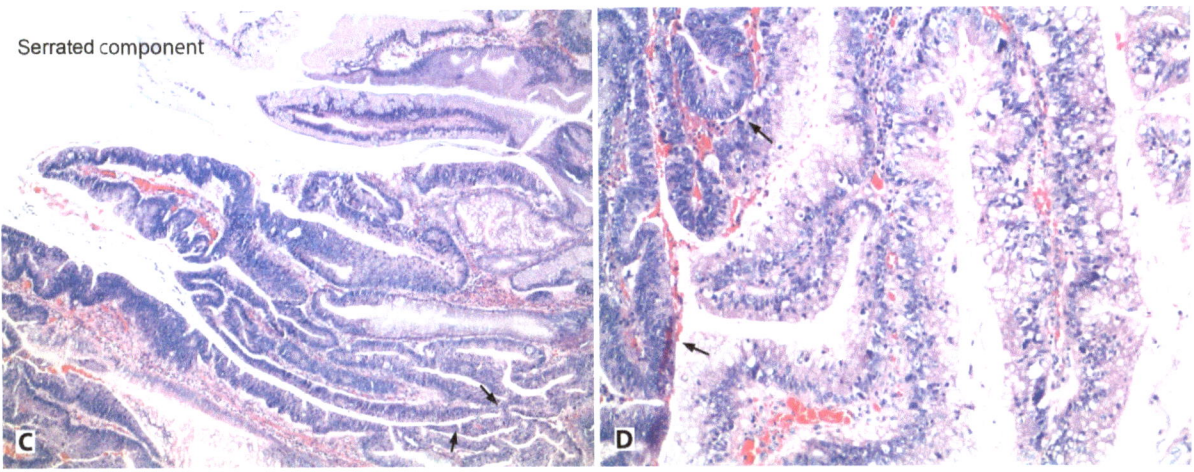

Figure 1.12 Sessile serrated adenoma (A & B) typical features of a serrated lesion, (C & D) note focus of intramucosal adenocarcinoma (arrows)

Villous Adenoma

Before the identification of villo-glandular polyp, colonic polyps were classified as hyperplastic polyp, adenomatous polyp or villous adenoma. The WHO classification is based on the fact that all colo-rectal adenomas possess both adenomatous and villous components with pure adenoma and villous adenoma forming the boundaries of the spectrum of adenomatous polyps of large bowel. However, pure villous adenoma has a high propensity of progression to adenocarcinoma as compared to tubular adenoma and tubulo-villous adenoma.

Gross appearance is distinct from that of a tubular adenoma and histologically tall villous projections supported by delicate stromal strands are seen (Figure 1.13 A, B). Some villous adenomas appear sessile but may also diffusely involve the recto-sigmoid mucosa in carpet like fashion spread over several centimeters. This latter will histologically show isolated tall villi arranged in linear pattern and may display invasive adenocarcinoma in the submucosa (Figure 1.13 C, D).

About 33% villous adenomas are suspected on per rectal examination [PR] and 90% can be reached and diagnosed on sigmoidoscopy. It can be as small as one cm or straddle 6-10 cm across the recto-sigmoid. Villous adenomas are by definition benign. They are direct precursors of adenocarcinoma and follow a cancerous temporal course unless interrupted by treatment. In one large series of 174 patients treated over a period of 1960 to1975, the duration of symptoms was 8 to 24 months. All recurrences occurred within 4- 5 years after treatment and 46 patients died during the follow up period (45). 23 benign adenomas had local excision and 50 patients with adenocarcinoma had resection. Whereas there is a positive correlation between size of the lesion and incidence of malignancy, even a small sized adenoma may show presence of invasive carcinoma. In fact, 36 patients with totally excised polyps harbored adenocarcinoma as seen on serially sectioned specimens. It is evident that villous adenomas are aggressive neoplasms with a rather high incidence of ensuing adenocarcinoma.

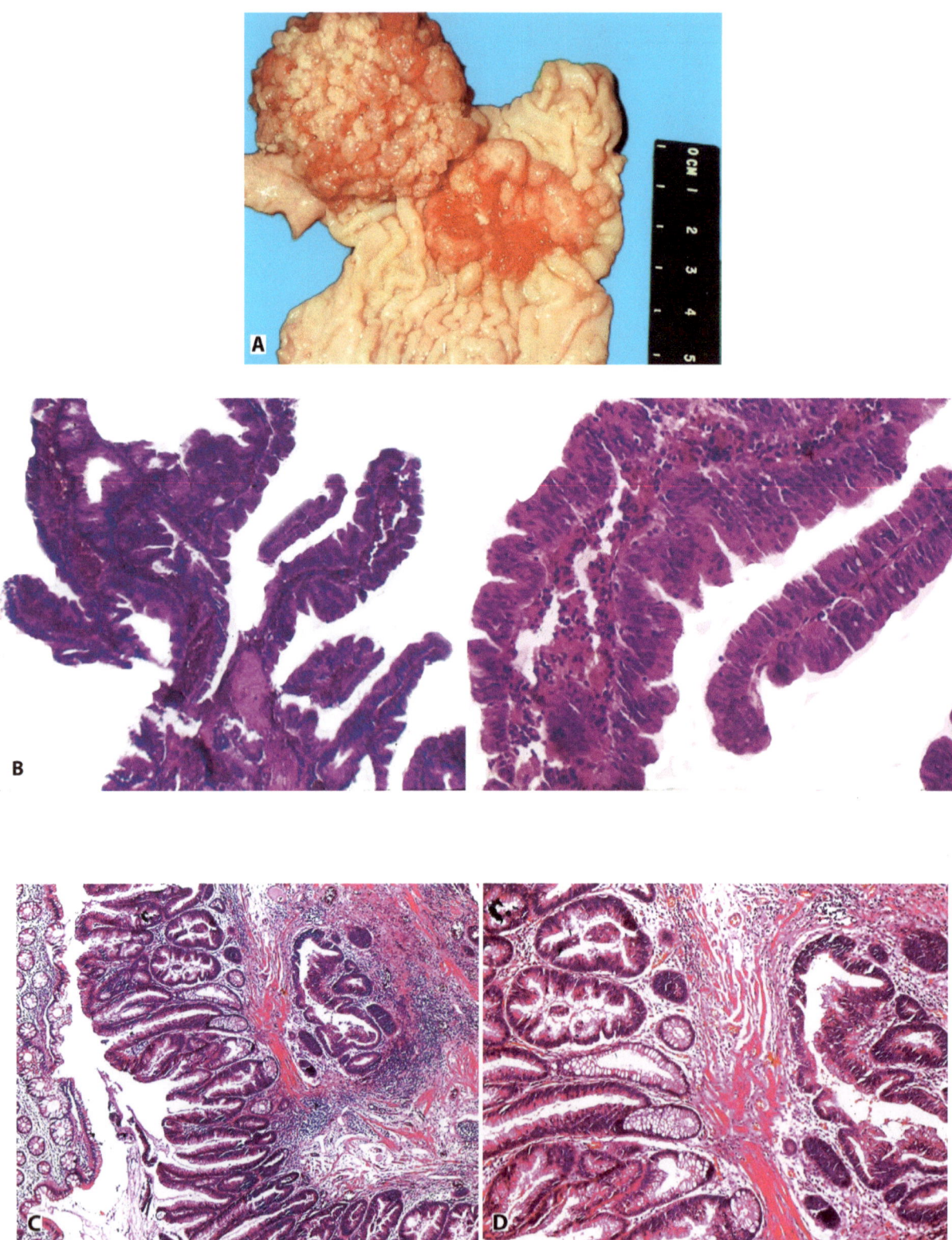

Figure 1.13 (A) Villous adenoma in a case of HNPCC, note large villous adenoma adjoining a centrally ulcerated invasive adenocarcinoma; (B) histologically the villous tumor appears benign, despite a large size of the resected adenoma (C & D) histology of invasive adenocarcinoma arising from villous adenoma

Miscellaneous Polypoid Lesions

Colitis cystica profunda

A rather rare condition characterized by epithelium-lined mucous cysts deep to the muscularis mucosae in the wall of rectum and colon (46). A localized type usually restricted to rectum, a diffuse form involving extensive parts of large bowel and a segmental form have been described. 60 cases are reported in a period of 1967-1981. This lesion has been encountered in association with colostomy sites, radiation induced strictures, SRUS and as misplaced epithelial nests in adenomatous polyps. Colitis cystica profunda is regarded as a regenerative phenomenon in which there is an on-going injury. Histologically, prominent glandular proliferation producing polypoid lesions is present. The glands show extensive cystic dilatation with pools of mucin incompletely lined by columnar epithelium. Many such glands extend deep in to muscularis mucosae mimic a well-differentiated adenocarcinoma (Figure 1.14 A, B, C). Marked acute and chronic inflammation is often seen around ruptured glands

In the past a fair number cases were misdiagnosed as mucin secreting well differentiated adenocarcinoma. The surgical pathologist should be well aware of this mimicry.

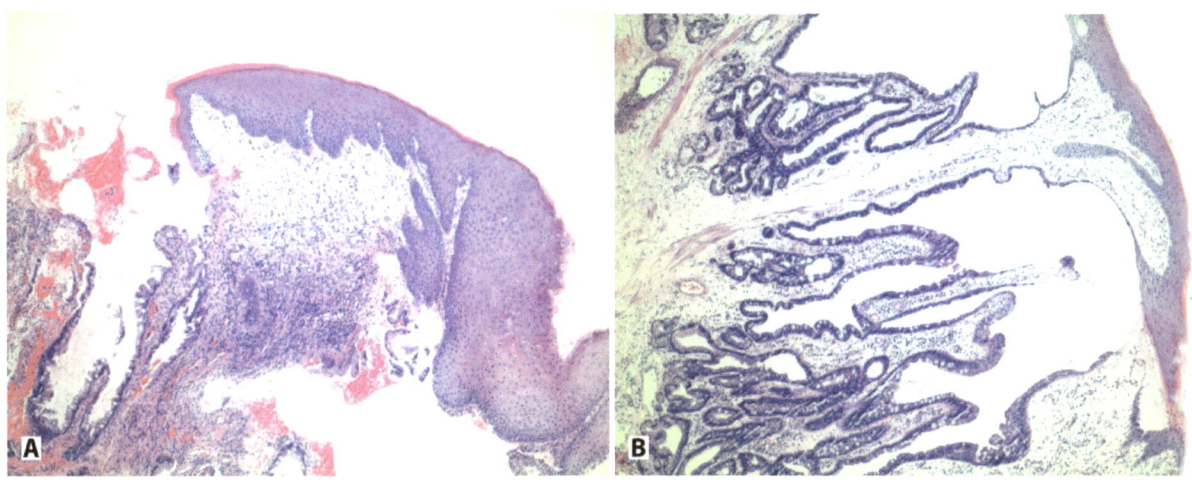

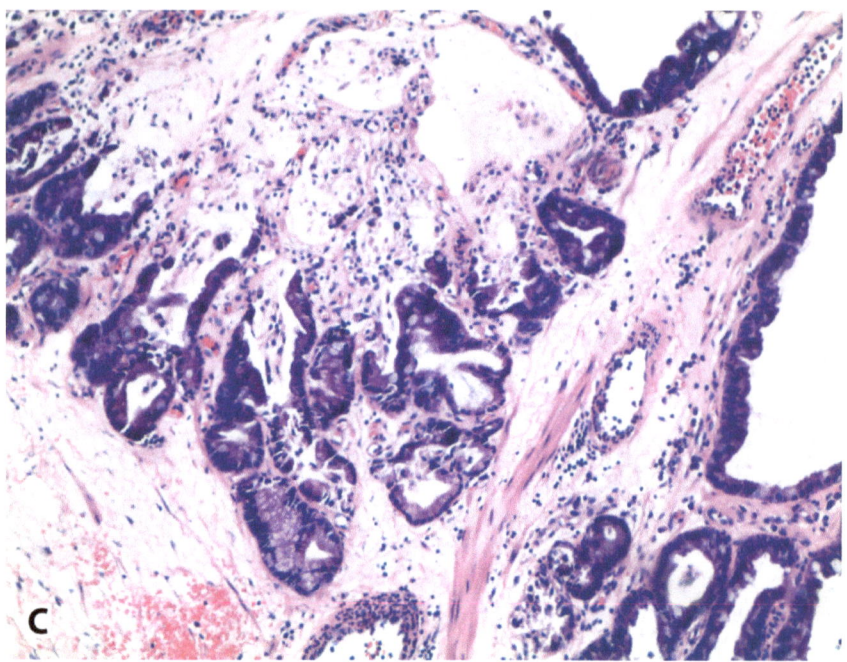

Figure 1.14 Colitis cystica profunda: a 45 year man complained of rectal bleeding and mass and the biopsy was interpreted as adenocarcinoma. (A & B) large elongated dilated & some cystic glands reaching beyond the level of muscularis mucosa with edema and inflammation; (C) thickened hyperchromatic crowded small to medium disoriented glands

Granular cell tumor

This small mucosal tumor, solitary or multiple is incidentally detected on endoscopy. It is benign and composed of large polygonal cells containing abundant PAS positive {not shown} granules and small uniform nuclei. (Figure 1.15 A, B, C) The cells express S-100 protein, suggesting a Schwannian differentiation (47).

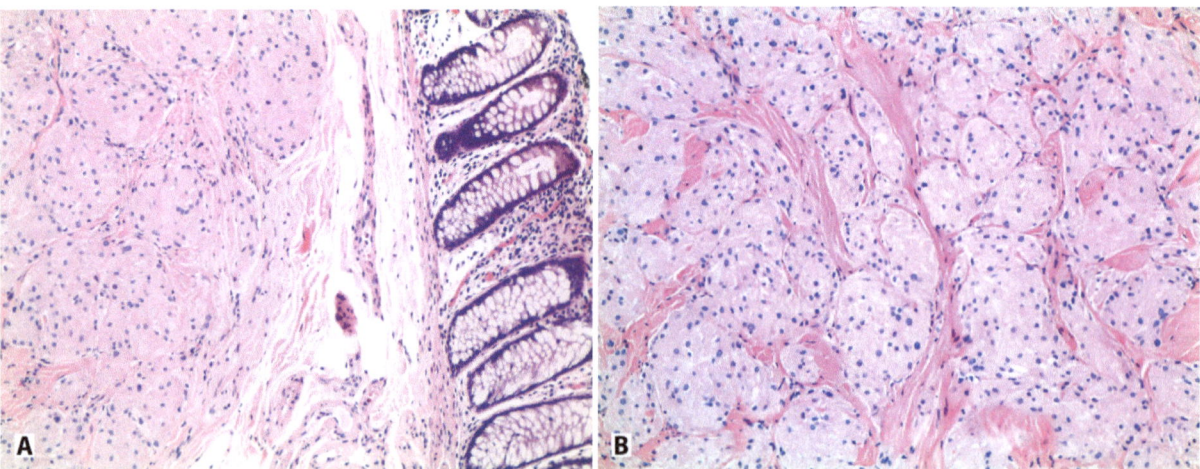

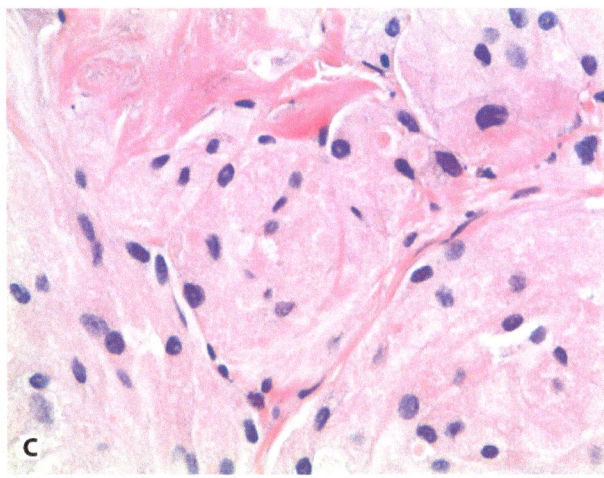

Figure 1.15 Granular cell tumor of colon: (A) colonic mucosa overlying circumscribed benign tumor, (B & C) large polygonal cells with copious cytoplasm rich in granules, and small uniform nuclei

Ganglioneuroma

The tumor has a predilection to occur in rectum and left colon. It usually presents as solitary 1 to 2 cm polyp or some times as multiple polyps. Diffuse murally occurring ganglioneuromas [ganglioneuromatosis] are frequent associated with NF1 and multiple endocrine neoplasia type 2b (48). Histologically, ill-defined whorls of small spindly Schwann cells and scattered ganglions cells are seen in the expanded lamina propria with intervening colonic glands (Figure 1.16 A, B, C, D). Ganglion cells show NSE and synaptophysin positivity and Schwann cells express S100 protein and often GFAP.

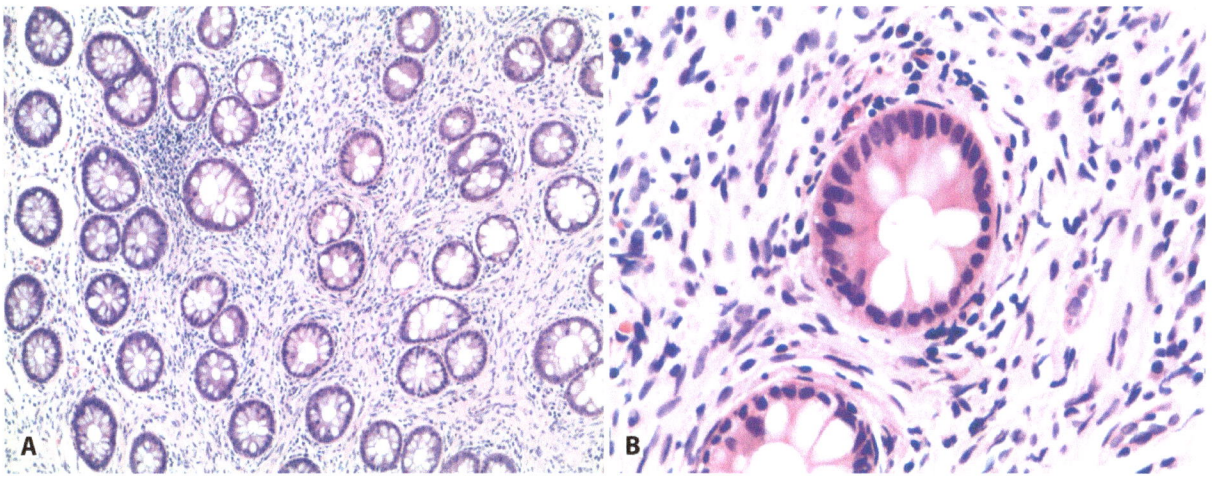

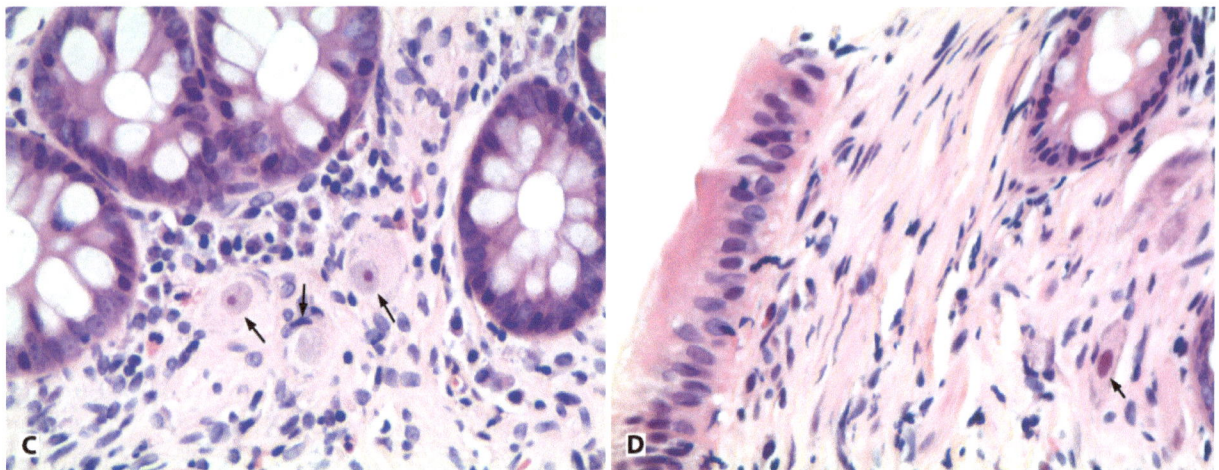

Figure 1.16 Ganglioneuroma: (A & B) whorls of short spindle shaped cells within lamina propria and arranged around glands, (C & D) ganglion cells (arrows)

Kaposi's sarcoma of GI tract:

According to a screening program conducted in the 1990s Kaposi's sarcoma occurred in 38% to 51% of patients having HIV/AIDS (49). In non-HIV state this tumor may exceptionally occur in GI tract. In most cases, stomach is commonly involved followed by colon. It is incidentally found as multiple small sub mucosal nodules. Colon may be involved simultaneously. Gastrointestinal bleeding may be the presenting finding in cases with large mural tumors (50). Histologically, the lesion is characterized by a hemorrhagic spindle cell proliferation with extravasation of red blood cells (Figure 1.17 A, B, C, D). Some tumor cells contain eosinophilic hyaline globules and immunohistochemical demonstration of herpes virus-8 (HHV-8) in the nuclei of tumor cells is diagnostic (51).

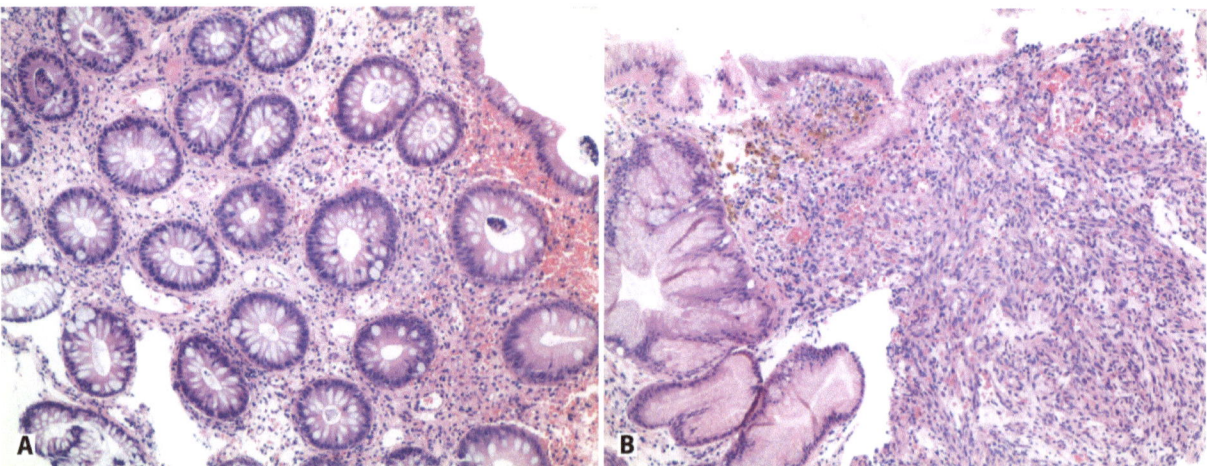

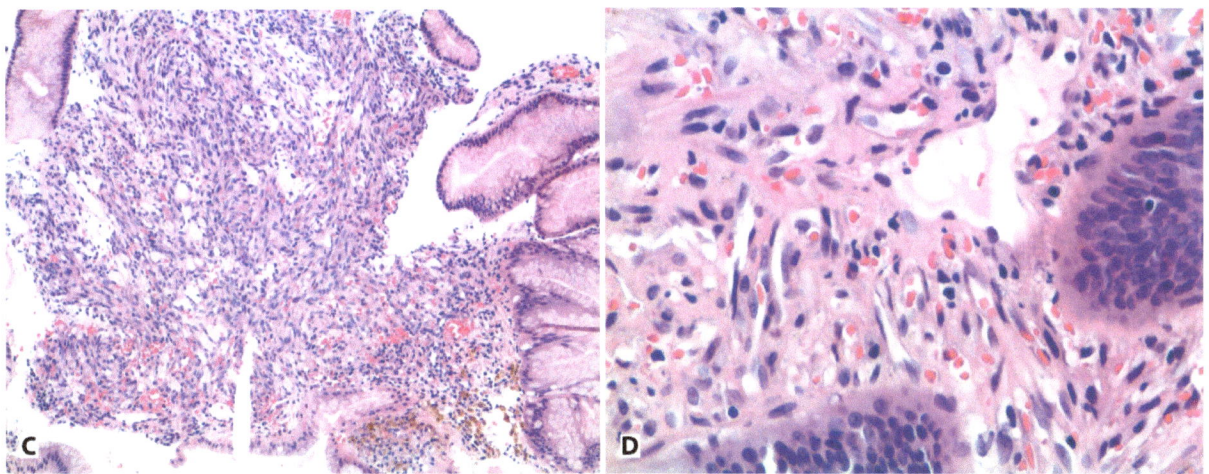

Figure 1.17 Kaposi's sarcoma of colon: (A) colonic mucosa shows cellular lamina propria and hemorrhages; (B & C) a cellular small spindle cell component with interstitial slit like capillaries containing RBCs (D) several isolated RBCs extravaseted in the spindly component

Gastrointestinal Polyposis Syndromes

Colorectal cancer (CRC) is one of the commonest cancers prevalent in large parts of the World. 2% to 5% of CRCs occur in the setting of well defined polyposis syndromes and about 30% exhibit increased familial risk most likely related to inheritance. The etiologies of these latter inherited CRCs are not completely understood. Most common among polyposis syndromes include: Lynch syndrome, familial adenomatous polyposis (FAP), and certain hamartomatous conditions like Peutz-Jeghers syndrome (polyposis).

With remarkable advances in the field of genetics, causative genes of several major hereditary GI polyposis syndromes have been discovered. There is a US government funded public medical genetics resource for health care and research available at no cost. The web site provides authoritative information on genetic testing and its use in diagnosis, management and genetic counseling. A precise understanding of genetics of inherited CRCs is important in identifying at-risk individuals, improving cancer surveillance and prevention strategies, and better diagnostic and therapeutic approaches. It can not be too strongly emphasized that the morbidity and mortality of cases of inherited CRCs has been considerably improved.

Heredity and Cololrectal Cancer

Facts:
- >1% Familial adenomatous Polyposis conventional and attenuated
- 3%-5% Hereditary Non-Polyposis Colorectal Cancer Syndrome
- 15%-20% Etiologies of these hereditary CRCs not completely understood

Classification of Hereditary GI polyposis Syndromes (Genes), inheritance

Familial adenomatous polyposis

- Adenomatous polyposis coli (APC), autosomal dominant inheritance
- Gardner syndrome (APC), autosomal dominant inheritance
- Turcot syndrome (APC), autosomal dominant inheritance

Hamartomatous polyposis

- Peutz-Jeghers syndrome (STK11), autosomal dominant inheritance
- Familial juvenile polyposis (SMAD4 or (BMPR1A), autosomal dominant inheritance
- Cowden's syndrome (PTEN), autosomal dominant inheritance
- Ruvalcaba -Myrthe-Smith-syndrome (PTEN), autosomal dominant inheritance

(Adapted from Bronner MP: Gastrointestinal Inherited Polyposis Syndromes. Mod Pathol 2003; 16: 359-365)

Hamartomatous Polyposis Syndromes:
(53, 54) Table 1.4

Disease	Genetics	Manifestations
Juvenile polyposis	SMAD4 OR BMPRIA	multiple polyps in GI tract (autosomal dominant)
Peutz-Jeghers	STK11	hamartomatous polyps, Muco-cutaneous pigmentation Increased risk of malignancy
Cowden syndrome	PTEN	Polyps throughout GI tract Fibroma, lipoma, hemangioma etc. Risk for breast, thyroid carcinoma
Bannayan-Riley-Ruvalcaba	PTEN	Polyps in colon and tongue
Hereditary Mixed Polyposis	CRAC 1	Classical adenoma, juvenile polyp, serrated Adenoma, hyperplastic polyp
Cronkhite –Canada	Non-hereditary	microencephaly, lipomas, juvenile Polyps in GI tract, diarrhea, cachexia

From the data above certain generalizations can be made:

1] The syndromes based on APC gene mutation are the most common and apart from CRCs many extra colonic manifestations, particularly emergence of carcinomas occur in other organs.

2] There is a very high incidence of carcinomas involving various parts of GI tract in Peutz-Jeghers syndrome, which harbor hamartomatous polyps, which do not themselves become malignant. This is partly true for other hamartomatous syndromes

3] In addition to various types of polyps of GI tract, benign mesenchymal tumors (osteoma, fibroma, lipoma, hemangioma etc) are commonly encountered in the hamartomatous polyposis syndromes (55, 56).

A fair number of these polyposis syndromes are exceedingly rare and even the most senior and very experienced surgical pathologists may not have encountered a single instance of some syndromes. It is not possible to do justice to all polyposis syndromes and only the relatively important ones will be described. There are 3 autosomal dominant inherited polyposis syndromes: familial adenomatous polyposis, juvenile polyposis and Peutz-Jeghers polyposis, which predispose to cancers, particularly colorectal. The next important is hereditary non-polyposis colorectal cancer syndrome (HNPCC). Uncovering the genetic background will provide genetic testing for the family members of an affected patient.

Familial Adenomatous Polyposis [FAP]

Synonyms: Adenomatous polyposis coli, Familial polyposis coli (57, 58)

Definition:

An autosomal dominant disease resulting from germ line mutation in APC gene in chromosome 5, is characterized by the development of tens to thousands of adenomatous polyps (Figure 1.18 A, B, C, D) throughout the large intestine during the second decade of life with occurrence of adenocarcinoma in the untreated cases.

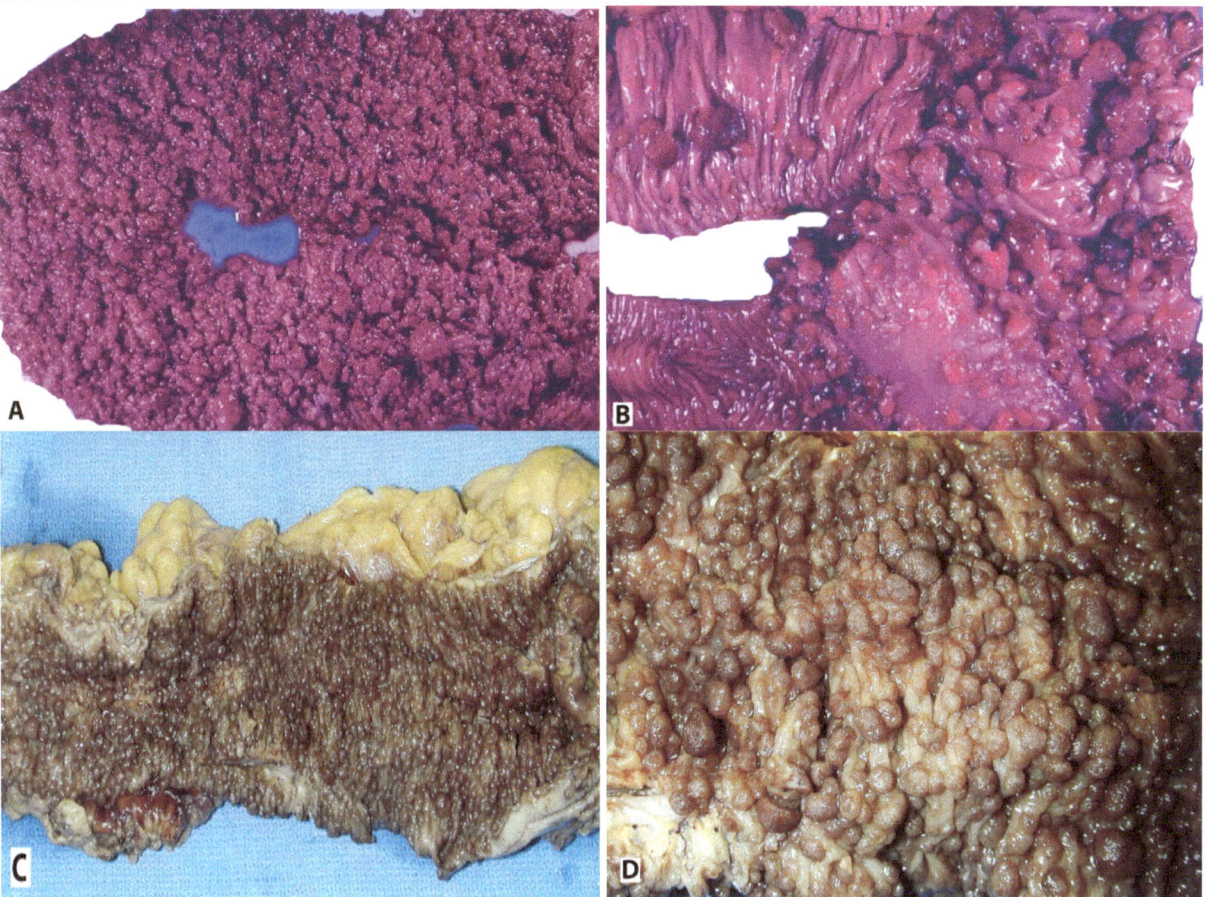

Figure 1.18 Familial adenomatous polyposis: (A& B) several thousands of closely packed 0.5 to 1cm polypoid tumors carpeting the colonic & rectal mucosa, (C & D) a second example of FAP

Clinical Findings:

Many patients remain asymptomatic for years unless there are large polyps causing bleeding or leading to severe symptomatic anemia. Cancer starts to develop about 1 decade after the appearance of polyps. Worldwide, about 80% to 85% of colorectal cancers are sporadic and approximately 15% to 20% familial with FAP accounting for 1% or so. There are other gastrointestinal manifestations: fundic gland polyps in stomach develop in 90% of FAP cases, adenomatous polyps in duodenum and ampulla of Vater, and adenomatous polyps in small intestine in few cases. This emphasizes the need to study almost entire GI tract on endoscopy.

Extra-intestinal Manifestations in FAP:

Extra-intestinal manifestations are common in hereditary colorectal cancer syndromes and particularly in FAP the lifetime risk of these lesions exceeds 30%. FAP is multisystem disorder of growth and has varied presentations:

Thyroid and pancreatic cancer
Hepatoblastoma
Medulloblastoma of cerebellum
Desmoid tumors and dental abnormalities
Various benign tumors such as adrenal adenoma, osteoma
Upper gastrointestinal polyps in FAP- located in stomach, duodenum, and periampullary region

In FAP syndromes benign fundic gland polyps [90% nonmalignant] and adenomatous polyps [10% malignant] often occur in stomach

Duodenal and ampulla of Vater adenomatous polyps are common manifestation of FAP and found in 30% to70% with life time risk reaching up to 100%. 70% of these polyps are of adenomatous type and ensuing adenocarcinoma is an important cause of death in cases of FAP The extra intestinal conditions are individually quite rare but collectively constitute a challenge to the physician in diagnosis and management of polyposis syndromes. With improved longevity from CRCs due to better prevention, extra-intestinal clinical problems will increase

Desmoid tumors in FAP

(Figure 1.19 A, B, C)

These slow growing mesenchymal tumors consist of fibroblasts and myofibroblasts in a rich fibrous matrix. They lack metastatic potential but display an aggressive local behavior with random and extensive infiltration in the surrounding structures. Nearly 80% occur in the abdomen and commonly involve small intestine and mesentery. Recurrence rate is high even after attempted wide local excision, and is attended by high mortality.

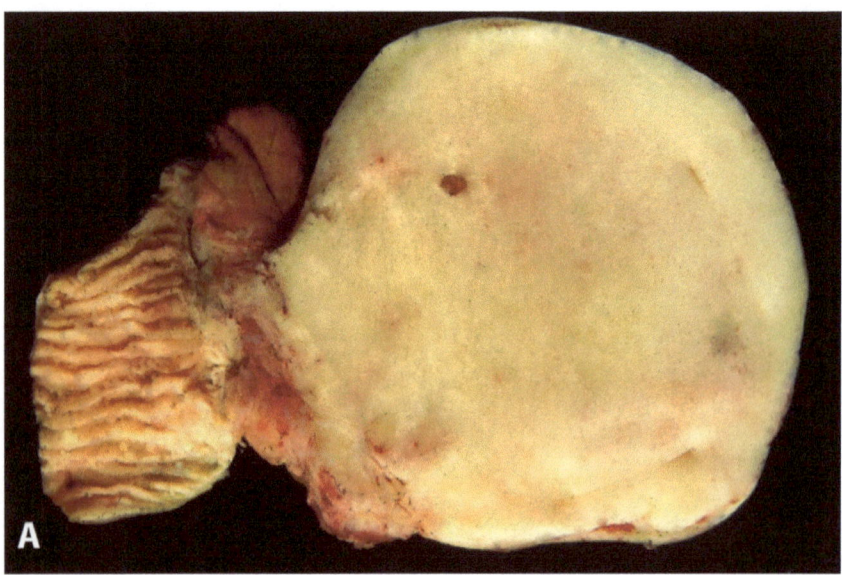

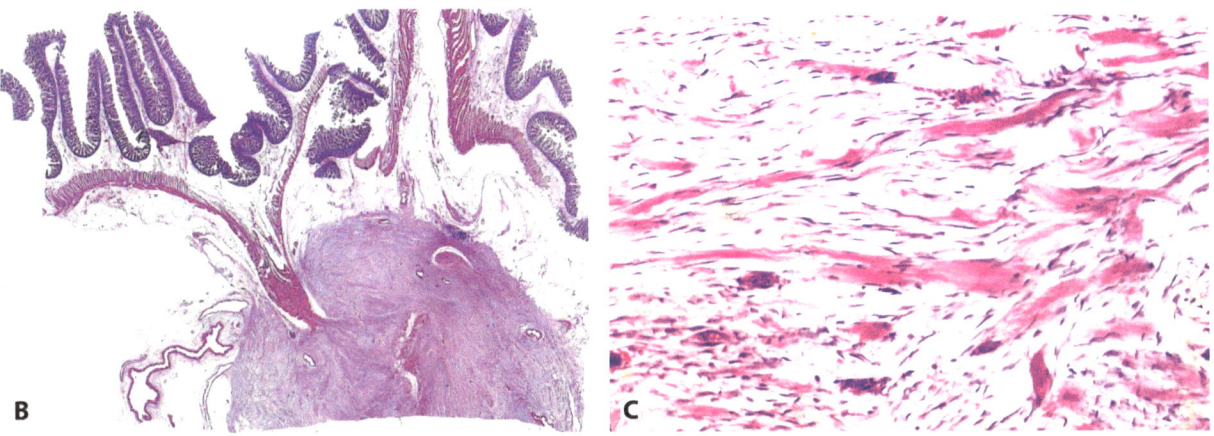

Figures 1.19 Desmoid tumors in FAP (A) a circumscribed whitish tumor of small bowel (B) tumor arising from muscularis propria and projecting into the mesentery; (C) fibrocollagenous tumor rich in bands of hyalinized collagen

Attenuated FAP (AFAP)

The attenuated form derives its name from greatly diminished number of polyps in these cases, averaging 30 adenomatous polyps in the colon. There is prominent variation in the numbers of these polyps in different patients but polyps are <100 as compared to thousands found in classical FAP. The colonic cancer develops much later in AFAP [about a decade] than in FAP. AFAP syndromes include Gardner's and Turcot's syndromes

Gardner's Syndrome

Discovered in 1962, the syndrome is characterized by the typical manifestations of FAP and the presence of osteomas, fibromas, and epidermoid cysts.

Turcot's Syndrome

Turcot's syndrome results from distinct germ line mutations in either the APC gene or the DNA mismatched repair genes (HNPCC). In this syndrome adenomatous polyposis is accompanied by cerebellar medulloblastoma. HNPCC/Turcot patients manifest adenomatous polyposis and Glioblastoma multiforme

Peutz-Jeghers Syndrome (PJS)

Definition

Gastrointestinal hamartomatous polyposis, mucocutaneous melanin pigmentation and high risk for a wide array of malignancies mostly arising from GI tract constitute PJS.

Clinical findings

PJS is an autosomal dominant condition with 50% of cases familial and 50% having new mutations. Most polyps are found in small intestine and others in stomach and colon. Melanosis typically occurs on the lips [>90%] and buccal mucosa [83%] (Figure 1.20 A). They are also seen on hands and feet. The polyps vary in size from microadenomas to polyps several cm long. The polyps may run into hundreds carpeting the mucosa or may be even be solitary (Figure 1.20 B) The polyps are made up of groups of near normal mucosal glands separated by thick bands of hypertrophic smooth muscle emanating from muscularis mucosae (Figure 1.20 C). This is typical hamartomtous presentation of the polyp.

PJS is a premalignant condition and carcinoma of GI tract is a frequent complication. Reports of carcinoma in PJS involving esophagus, stomach, small bowel and colon have appeared in the literature. However, most carcinomas in PJS have not originated from the hamartomatous polyps. Adenocarcinomas commonly occur in pancreas, lung and breast. A rare benign ovarian tumor, called sex cord tumor with annular tubules (SCTAT) has been reported in most female patients harboring the stigmata of PJS.

Microscopic

Peutz-Jeghers polyps are composed of normal histological elements belonging to the site in which they arise, indeed a true hamartoma. Histologically, these polyps display frond like architecture and consist of stratified mucosal glands [crypts] with normal lining cells, supported by bands of smooth muscle emanating from muscularis mucosae (Figure 1.21 A, B). PJP is the most common polyp among the hamartomatous polyposis family and is inherited as an autosomal dominant trait with variable penetrance, like the rest. In 20% to 50% of patients family history can be elicited. The polyps consist of scattered cystic glands lined by normal appearing goblet cells, the surface epithelium is ulcerated and lamina propria variably inflamed. The polyps are larger than their counterpart sporadic ones. A rare benign ovarian tumor, called sex cord tumor with annular tubules) (Figure 1.21 C, D), has been reported in most female patients harboring the stigmata of PJS. Grossly, multiple pedunculated polyps are seen in all cases and can be found in stomach, small intestines and large intestines. Not uncommonly large solitary lobulated white pink polyp is seen (Figure 1.21 A)

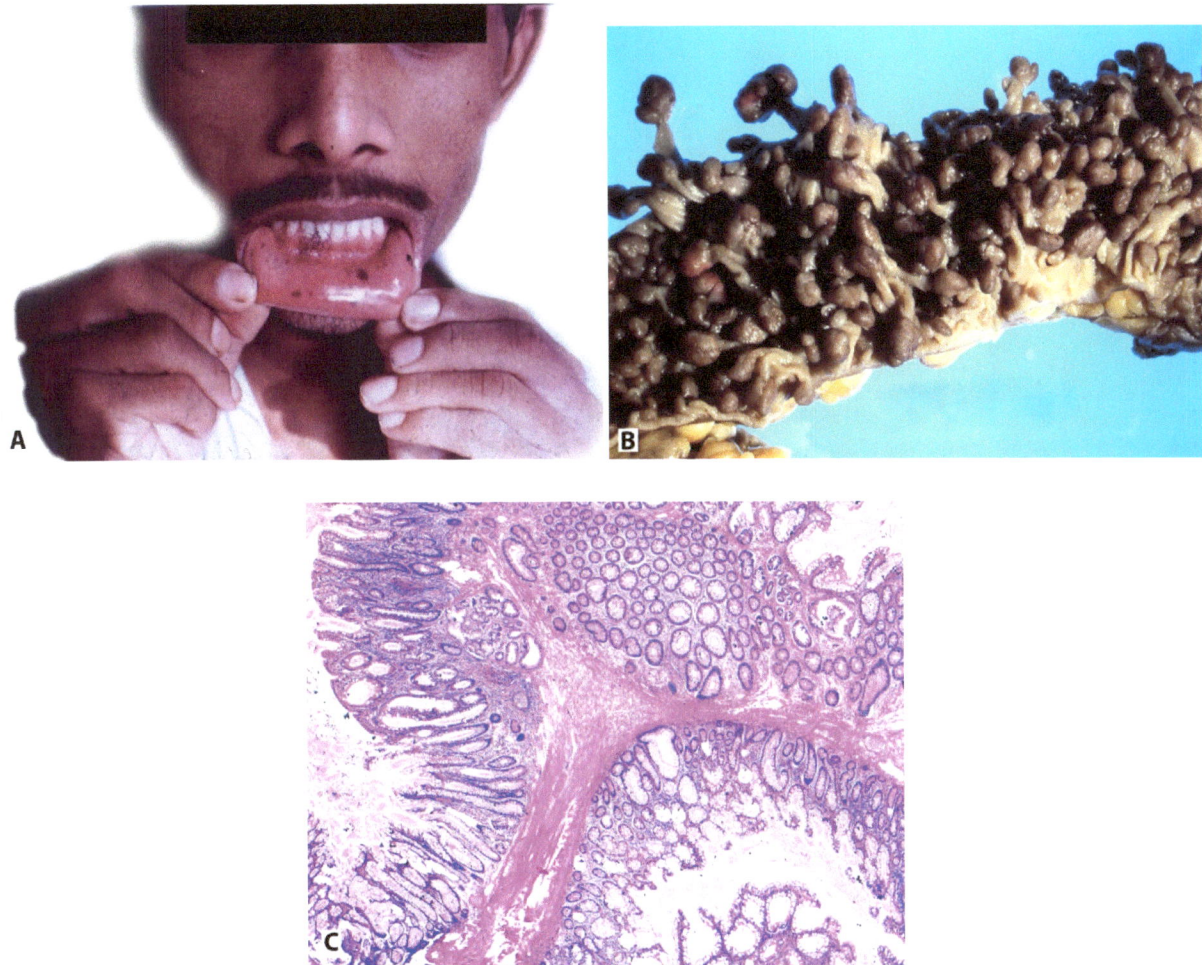

Figure 1.20 Peutz-Jeghers syndrome: (A) black spots on lower lip of this 25 year male having symptoms of intestinal obstruction (B) multiple pedunculated polyps in small bowel (C) The polyp consists of normal mucosal glands and few villi and three bands of smooth muscle emanating from muscularis mucosa.

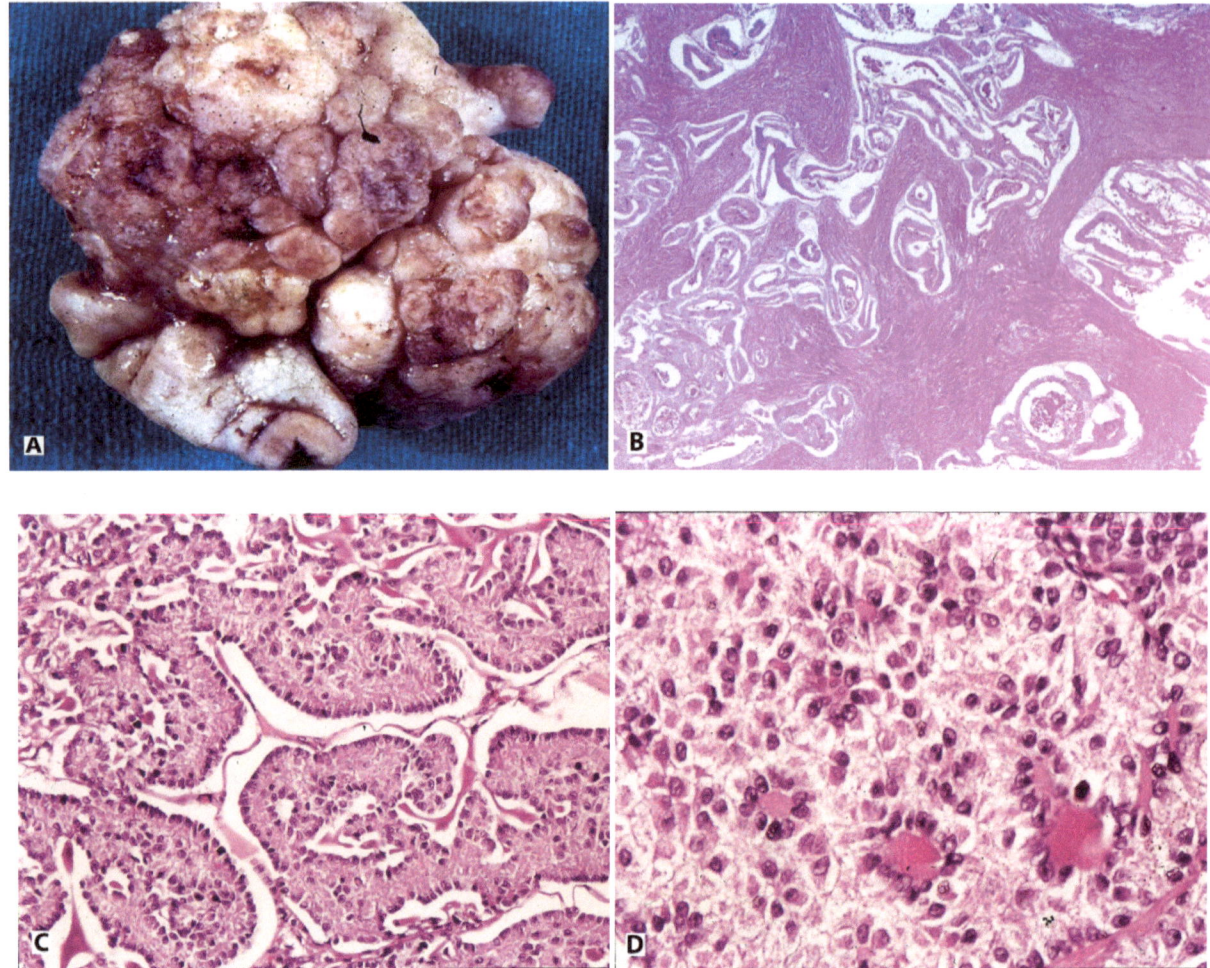

Figure 1.21 Peutz-Jeghers Syndrome (A) a large multinodular polyp from sigmoid colon (B) the polyp consists of islands of colonic glands separated by thick hypertrophic fascicles of smooth muscle (C & D) low and high power pictures of sex cord tumor with annular tubules (SCTAT) in this 15 year old adolescent girl

Juvenile Polyposis Syndrome (JPS)

It is well established that JPS patients are at a very high risk for development of gastrointestinal adenocarcinoma, usually colorectal carcinoma and risk ranging from 20% to 70%. All juvenile polyps should be carefully examined to rule out dysplasia because cancer in JPS arises from neoplastic transformation of the polyp itself, unlike in PJS.

Solitary juvenile polyp is fairly common lesion and occurs typically in rectum in children and adolescents. The polyp is ulcerated and often pedunculated. It consists of hyperplastic glands, scattered cystic glands, acutely inflamed lamina propria (Figure 1.22 A, B). The juvenile polyposis syndrome is characterized by the appearance of multiple polyps in the gastrointestinal tract, usually in a child, adolescent or young adult. Majority of the polyps found in Juvenile Polyposis Syndrome are non-neoplastic, hamartomatous, self-limiting and benign, but there is an increased risk of adenocarcinoma.

The World Health Organization criteria for diagnosis of juvenile polyposis syndrome are:

1. More than five juvenile polyps in the colon or rectum (Figure 1.23 A, B)

2. Juvenile polyps throughout the gastrointestinal tract; or
3. Any number of juvenile polyps in a person with a family history of juvenile polyposis.

Age at onset is variable. The term 'Juvenile' in the title of Juvenile Polyposis Syndrome refers to the histological type of the polyps rather than age of onset. Affected individuals may present with rectal bleeding, abdominal pain, diarrhea or anemia. The polyps can be sessile or pedunculated.

Lifetime risk of developing cancers of the gastro-intestinal tract in people with Juvenile Polyposis Syndrome ranges from 9% to 50%. Juvenile Polyposis Syndrome can occur sporadically in families or be inherited in an autosomal dominant manner. Solitary polyps have no significant risk of cancer. But multiple polyps (>5), polyposis syndrome of the colon carry a 10% risk of developing into cancer. This is mainly because of juvenile polyps developing adenomatous tissue.

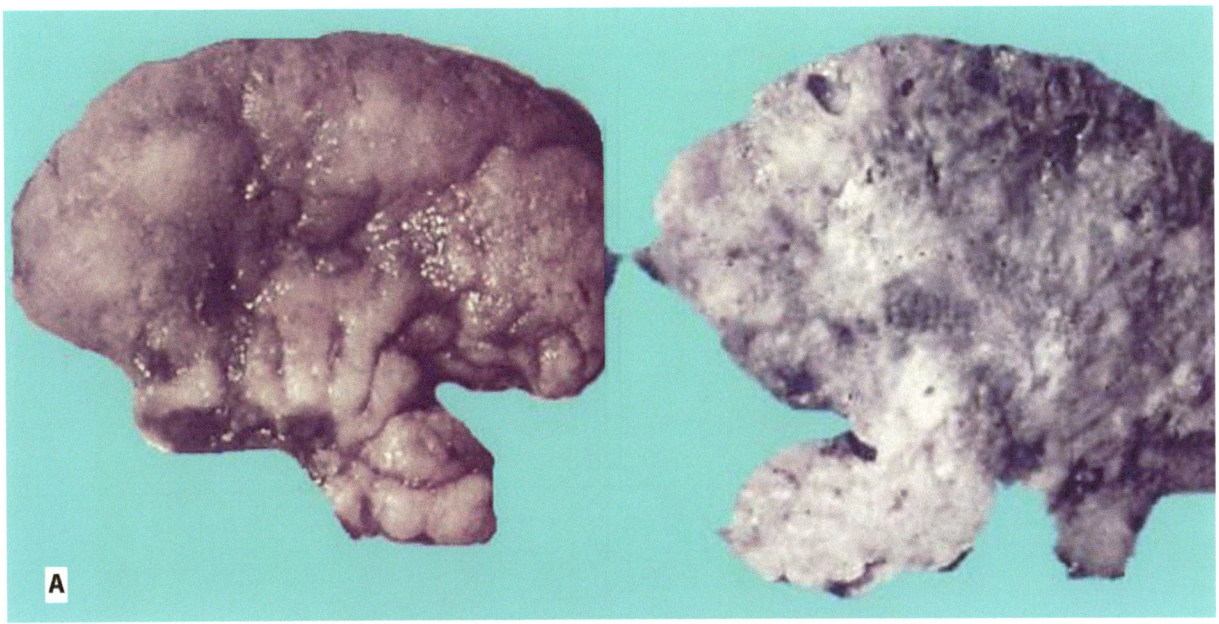

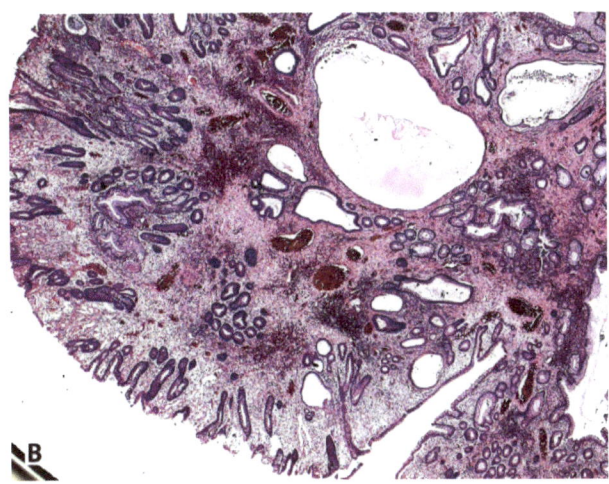

Figure 1.22 Solitary juvenile polyp of rectum: (A) external surface of pedunculated polyp, note fine cystic spaces (glands) on the sectioned surface; (B) histology showing scattered cystic glands of variable sizes and expanded inflammatory lamina propria

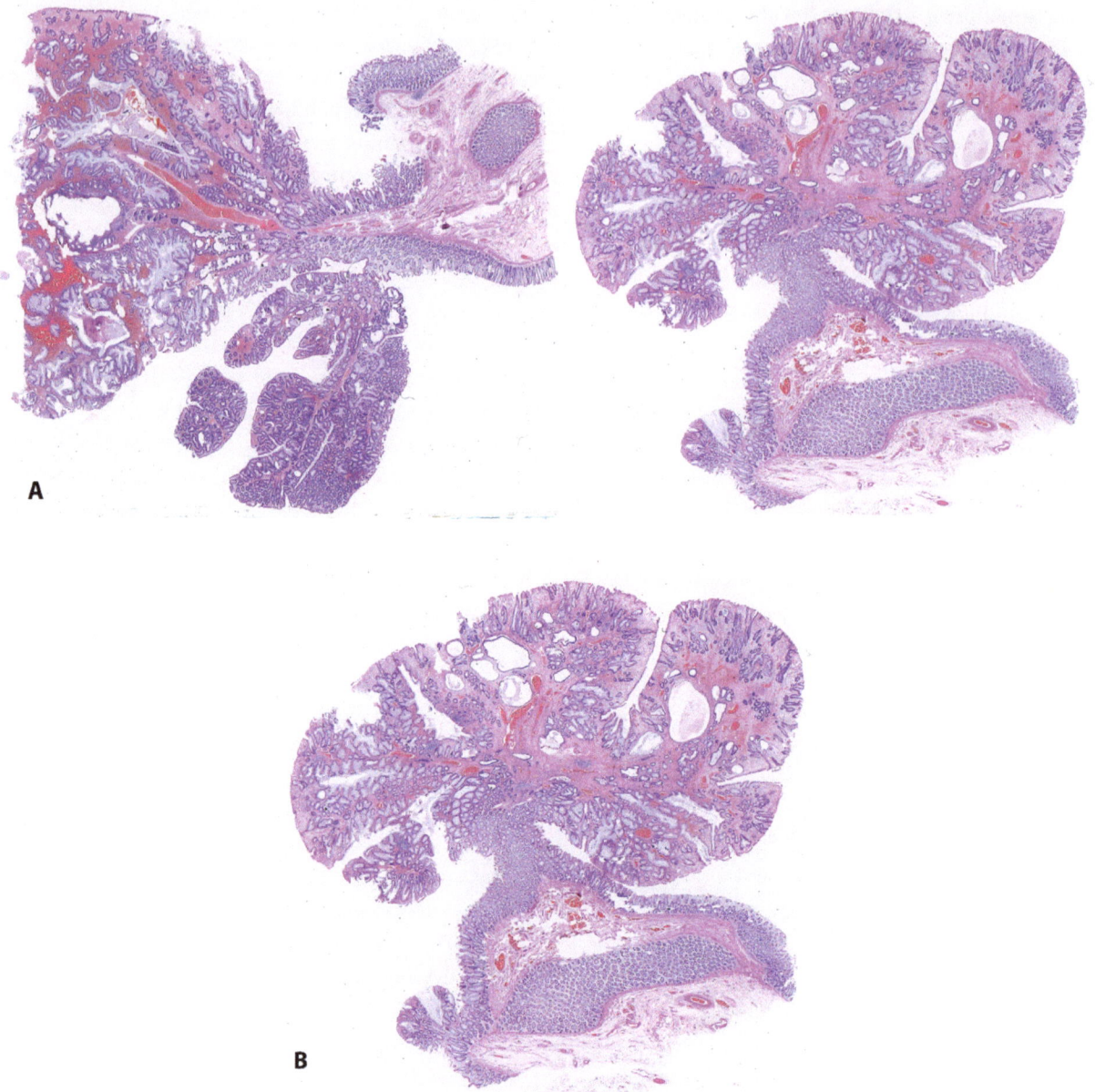

Figure 1.23 (A) A case of juvenile polyposis syndrome: multiple and branching juvenile polyps with typical morphology as seen on whole mount section (B) some more polyps in the same case

Hereditary Non-polyposis Colorectal Cancer (HNPCC)

Definition

HNPCC also termed Lynch Syndrome (LS) (58) is inherited in an autosomal dominant fashion and is caused by inherited defects in at least one of a family of DNA mismatch repair enzymes (HMSH 1Hmhs 2, Hmsh 6, Hpms 2). The syndrome accounts for 2 % to 5% of all CRC cases.

Clinical findings

The risk of colonic cancer is 80% to 90% in the affected patient and that for endometrium 40% to 60%, stomach 11-19% and Ovary 9%. Several tools are available to assist clinical diagnosis of Lynch syndrome including analyses of family history, tumor testing, mutation prediction models and genetic testing. It is important to obtain a detailed personal and family history. Amsterdam Criteria II and Revised Bethesda Guidelines are used in clinical practice to identify individuals at risk for Lynch syndrome.

Amsterdam Criteria II

At least three relatives with colorectal, endometrial, small bowel, ureter, or renal pelvis cancer; all of the following must be met:
- One affected individual is a first degree relative of the other two
- At least two successive generations affected
- At least one tumor diagnosed before the age of 50 years
- Familial adenomatous polyposis has been excluded

Revised Bethesda Guidelines

Requires at least one of the following:
- CRC diagnosed in a patient who is less than 50 years of age
- Presence of synchronous, metachronous CRC, or other LS-associated tumors, regardless of age
- CRC diagnosed in a patient who is less than 60 years of age with MSI-H histology
- CRC diagnosed in an individual and one or more first degree relatives with an LS-associated tumor with at least one of the cancers being diagnosed under age 50 years
- CRC diagnosed in an individual and two or more first or second degree relatives with LS-associated tumors, regardless of age

Pathology

Colon cancers and polyps arise in Lynch syndrome at a younger age of onset and more proximal in location compared to sporadic neoplasms. Histologically, cancers are often poorly differentiated, mucinous, and characterized by a high level of microsatellite instability.

References of polyps

1. Carmack SW, Genta RM, Schuler CM, et al. The current spectrum of gastric polyps: a 1-year national study of over 120.000 patients. Am J Gastroenterol. 2009;104:1524-1532
2. Gencosmanoglu R, Sen-Oran E, Kurtkaya-Yapicier O, et al: Gastric polypoid lesions: Analysis of 150 endoscopic polypectomy specimens from 91 patients. World J Gastroenterol 2003; 9:2236-2239.
3. Abraham SC, Singh VK, Yardley JH, et al: Hyperplastic polyps of the stomach: Associations with histologic patterns of gastritis and gastric atrophy. Am J Surg Pathol 2001; 25:500-507.
4. Ljubicic N, Banic M, Kujundzic M, et al: The effect of eradicating Helicobacter pylori infection on the course of adenomatous and hyperplastic gastric polyps. Eur J Gastroenterol Hepatol 1999; 11:727-730.
5. Gonsalez-Obeso E, Fugita WH, Deshpande V, et al. Gastric hyperplastic polyps: a heterogeneous clinico-pathologic group including a distinct subset best categorized as mucosal prolapse polyp. Am J Surg Pathol 2011; 35:67--677
6. Abraham SC, Nobukawa B, Giardielo FM et al. Fundic gland polyps in familial adenomatous polyposis: Neoplasms with frequent somatic adenomatous polyposis coli gene alterations Am J Pathol 2000;157:747-754.
7. Bulow S, Lauritsen KB, Johansen A et al. Gastroduodenal polyps in familial adenomatous coli. Dis Colon Rectum 1985; 28:90-93

8. Burt RW: Gastric fundic gland polyps. Gastroenterology 2003; 125:1462-1469.

9. Choudhry U, Boyce Jr HW, Coppola D: Proton pump inhibitor-associated gastric polyps: A retrospective analysis of their frequency, and endoscopic, histologic, and ultrastructural characteristics. Am J Clin Pathol 1998; 110:615-621.

10. Ming SC, Goldman H: Gastric polyps: A histogenetic classification and its relation to carcinoma. Cancer 1965; 18:721-729.

11. OberhuberG, Stolte M. Gastric polyps: an update of their pathology and biological significance. Virchow's Arch. 2000; 427: 581-590

12. Abraham SC, Montgomery EA, Singh VK, et al: Gastric adenomas: Intestinal-type and gastric-type adenomas differ in the risk of adenocarcinoma and presence of background mucosal pathology. Am J Surg Pathol 2002; 26:1276-1285.

13. Kamiya T, Morishita T, Asakura H, et al: Long-term follow-up study on gastric adenoma and its relation to gastric protruded carcinoma. Cancer 1982; 50:2496-2503.

14. Tan YM, Wong WK: Giant Brunneroma as an unusual cause of upper gastrointestinal hemorrhage: Report of a case. Surg Today 2002; 32:910-912.

15. Cassar-Pullicino VN, Davies AM, Hubscher S, et al: The nodular duodenum in chronic renal failure. Clin Radiol 1990; 41:326-330

16. Chatelain D, Maillet E, Boyer L, et al: Brunner gland hamartoma with predominant adipose tissue and ciliated cysts. Arch Pathol Lab Med 2002; 126:734-735.

17. Akino K, Kondo Y, Ueno A, et al: Carcinoma of duodenum arising from Brunner's gland. J Gastroenterol 2002; 37:293-296.

18. Brookes MJ, Manjunatha S, Allen CA, et al: Malignant potential in a Brunner's gland hamartoma. Postgrad Med J 2003; 79:416-41

19. Shimer GR, Helwig EB. Inflammatory fibroid polyps of the intestine. Am J Clin Pathol. 1984;81708-714

20. Kolodoziejczy KP, Yao T, Tsuneyoshi MInflammatory fibroid polyp of stomach. A special reference to an immunohistochemical profile of 42 cases Am J Surg Pathol 1993; 17:1159-1168

21. Pantanowitz L, Antonioli D, Pinkus GA et al. Inflammatory Fibroid Polyp of the gastrointestinal tract : evidence for a dendritic cells origin. Am J Surg Pathol 2004; 28:107-114

22. Imperiale TF, Wagner DR, Lin CY, et al. Results of screening colonoscopy among persons 40 to 49 years of age. N Engl J Med 2002;346:1781-178523. Fossi S, Bazzoli F, Ricciardiello L et al. Incidence and recurrence rates of colorectal adenomas in first degree asymptomatic relatives of patient with colon cancer. Am J Gastroenterol 2001;96:1601-1604

24 Winawer SJ, Zauber AG, Gerdes H, et al Risk of colorectal cancer in the families of patients with adenomatous polyps. National Polyp Study Workgroup. N Engl.J Med 1996; 334:1339-1340

25. Aitken JF, Bain CJ, Waard M, et al. Risk of colorectal adenomas in patients with a family history of colorectal cancer: some implications for screening programs. Gut;39:105-108

26. Winawer SJ, Zauber AG, Fletcher RH, et al. Guidelines for colonoscopy surveillance after polypectomy : A consensus update by the US Multi-Society Task Force on colorectal cancer and the American Cancer Society. Gastroenterology 2006; 130:1872-1885

27.Euscher ED, Niemann TH, Lucas JG et el. Large colorectal adenomas: An approach to pathologic evaluation. Am J Clin Pathol. 2001; 116:336-340

28. Yang G, Zheng W, Sun QR, et al. Pathologic features of initial adenomas as predictors for metachronous adenomas of the rectum. J Natl Cancer Inst 1998; 90:1661-1665

29. Loeve F, van Ballegooijen M, Boer R, et al. Colorectal cancer risk in adenoma patients: A nation-wide study. Int J Cancer 2004:111:147-151

30. Shinya H, Wolff WI. Morphology, Anatomic distribution and Cancer Potential of Colonic Polyps: An analysis of 7,000 Polyps Endoscopically Removed. Annals of Surg. 1979; 190: 679-683

31. Bussey HJR. Multiple Adenomas and Carcinomas. In Morson BC.(Ed) The pathogenesis of Colorectal Cancer. Philadelphia, W.B. Saunders & Co, 1978

32. Huang CS, O'obrien MJ, Yang S, et al. Hyperplastic polyps, serrated adenomas and serrated polyp neoplasia pathway. Am J Gastroenterol 2004; 99:2242-2255

33. Kearney J, Giovannucci E, Rimm EB, et al. Diet alcohol and smoking and the occurrence of polyps of the colon and rectum (United States). Cancer Causes Control. 1995; 6:45-56

34. Torlakovic E, Skuvlund E, Snover D et al. Morphological reappraisal of serrated colorectal polyps. Am J Surg Pathol 2003; 27:65-81

35. Estrada RG, Spjut HJ. Hyperplastic polyps of the large bowel. Am J Surg Pathol 1980;4:127-133

36. Jass JR. Hyperplastic polyps and colorectal cancer; Is there a link? Clin Gastroenterol Hepatol 2004; 2:1-8

37. Chung SN, Chen YT, Panczykiowski A, et al. Serrated Polyps With "Intermediate Features" of Sessile Serrated Polyp and Microvesicular Hyperplastic Polyp: a Practical Approach to the classification of Nondysplastic Serrated Polyps

38. Longacre TA, Fenoglio-Preiser CM. Mixed Hypoerplastic Adenomatous Polyps/Serrated Adenomas: A Distinct form of Colorectal Neoplasia. Am J Surg Pathol. 1990; 14: 524-537

39. Snover DC. Serrated polyps of the large intestine. Semin Diagn Pathol. 2005; 22:301-308

40. Oh K, Redston M, Odze RD. Support for hMLH1 and MGMT silencing as a mechanism of tumorigenesis in the hyperplastic-adenoma-carcinoma (serrated) carcinogenic pathway in the colon. Hum Pathol 2005; 36:101-111

41. Jass JR, Baker K, Zlobeck I, et al. Advanced colorectal polyps with molecular and morphological features of serrated polyps and adenomas: Concept of a "fusion" pathway to colorectal cancer. Histopathology 2006; 49:121-131

42. Snover DC, Jass JR, Fenoglio-Preiser C, et al. Serrated polyps of the large intestine: A morphologic and molecular review of an evolving concept. Am J Clin Pathol 2005; 124:380-391

43. Matsumoto T, Mizuno M, Shimizu M, et al. Serrated adenoma of the colorectum: Colonoscopic and histologic features. Gastrointest Endosc 1999; 49:736-742

44. Yantiss RK, Oh KY, Chen YT, et al. Filliform serrated adenomas: a clinicopathological, DNA ploidy, and immunohistochemical study of 18 cases. Am J Surg Pathol 2007; 31:1238-1245

45. Christiansen J, Kirkegaard, Ibsen J. Prognosis after treatment of villous adenoma of colon and rectum. Ann Surg. 1979; 189:404-408

46. Schein M, Vetter M, Decker GAG. Colitis cystica profunda simulating rectal carcinoma S Afr Med J. 1987; 72: 289-290

47. Melo CR, Melo IS, Schmitt FC, et al.Multicentric granular cell tumor of colon: report of a patient with 2 tumors. Am J Gastroenterol 1993; 881785-1787

48. Shekika KM, Sobin LH. Ganglioneuroma of the gastrointestinal tract. Relation to von Recklinghausen disease and other multiple tumor syndrome. Am J Surg Pathol 1994; 18-250-257

49. Parente F, Cemuschi M, Orlando G, et al. Kaposi's sarcoma and AIDS: frequency of gastrointestinal involvement and its effects on survival. A prospective study in a heterogenous population. Scand J Gastoenterol. 1991; 26:1007-1012

50. Ravera M, Reggioei A, Cocozza E, et al. Kaposi's sarcoma and AIDS in Uganda: its frequency and gastroinestinal distribution. 1994 Ital J Gastroenterol 26:329-333

51. Kahl P, Buettner R, Frideriches N, et al. Kaposi's sarcoma of gastroentestinal tract: report of two cases and review of the literature Pathol Res Pract. 2007; 203: 227-231

References: Gastrointestinal Polyposis Syndromes

52 Bronner MP: Gastrointestinal Inherited Polyposis Syndromes. Mod Pathol 2003; 16: 359-365

53 Gammon A, Jasperson K, Kohlmann W, et al: Hamartomatous Polyposis Syndromes. Best Pract Res Clin gastroenterol. 2009; 23: 219-231

54 Calva D, Howe JR: Hamartomatous Polyposis Syndromes. Surg Clin North Am 2008; 88: 779

55 Groen EJ, Roos A, Muntinghe FL, et al: Extra-intestinal Manifestations of Familial Adenomatous Polyposis: Annals of Surgical Oncology 2008; 15: 2439-2450

56 Anaya DA, Chang GJ, Rodriguez-Bigas MA: Extracolonic Manifesttions of Hereditary Colorectal Cancer Syndromes. Clinics Clinics in Colon and Rectal Surgery 2008; 21: 263-270

57 Half E, Bercowich D, Rozen P: Familial Adenomatous Polyposis. Orphanet Journal of Rare Diseases. 2009; 4: 22

58 Jasperson KW, Tuohy TM, Necklason D, Burt RW: Hereditary and Familial Colon Cancer. Gastroenterology 2010; 138: 2044-2058

Malignant Lymphoma of Gastrointestinal Tract

Extranodal Lymphoma

Lymphomas arising in extranodal sites are intriguing. The types of lymphoma encountered vary widely from one extranodal site to another. The most common primary site of extranodal lymphoma is the gastrointestinal tract, accounting for 46% of lymphomas from all anatomical sites in the Author's experience [n=720] (Table 2.1). In our series of 335 GI tract lymphomas (Table 2.2), the most common organs involved were small intestines (89 cases) and stomach (80 cases) In a German multicenter study of 371 cases of gastrointestinal lymphoma, 74.8% lymphomas occurred in stomach, 8.6% in small intestine, 7.0% in ileo-cecal region and 6.5% in multiple sites in gastrointestinal tract. The distribution of histological subtypes in this series include DLBCL 59 cases (14 with MALT component and 45 without), MALT lymphoma of marginal zone type in 38 cases and 3 other cases (Follicular, mantle cell and peripheral T cell) (59).

The occurrence of a primary lymphoma in this system is often associated with a variety of predisposing factors like infection, immunodeficiency state, coeliac disease, chronic inflammatory bowel disease and immunosuppression after solid organ transplantation. These factors relate to various infections, namely: Helicobacter Pylori, HIV, Campylobacter Jejuni, EB virus, and human T cell lymphotropic virus-(HTLV-1).

It is necessary to differentiate primary gastrointestinal lymphoma from those associated with disseminated lymph nodal lymphoma. The accepted criteria for a diagnosis of primary gastrointestinal lymphoma include: absence of peripheral or mediastinal lymphadenopathy, normal differential and total WBC count, predominance of lymphoma in bowel and lack of involvement of liver and spleen (60).

Table 2.1: Sites of Extra-Nodal Lymphomas n = 720 Author's series [1970-2009]	
GI Tract	335
Skeletal System: [spine 67 + other 48]	115
Nervous System: [PCNSL 23 Cord 27 Orbit 20]	070
Soft Tissues	060
Skin: [NHL 22, MF 18]	040
Respiratory System: [Sino-nasal 22, Lung 8]	030
Others	069

** [Testis 41, Breast 10, Thyroid 10, Kidney 4, FGS 3, Adrenal 1]

Table 2.2 Lymphomas of GI Tract n = 335 Author's series [1970-2009]	
Oro-pharynx + Nasopharynx	42
Tonsils	61
Salivary Glands	16
Stomach	80
Small Intestines	89
Colo-Rectal [Right:Left = 34:13]	47

Malignant Lymphoma of Stomach

Mucosa-associated lymphoid tissue lymphoma and diffuse large B-cell lymphoma (DLBCL) account for 90% of all gastric lymphomas. DLBCL may have MALT component histologically or may arise de novo, i.e. without MALT component. Other histological types of lymphomas occurring in the stomach are mantle cell lymphoma, follicular lymphoma and Burkitt's lymphoma. These are identical to their counterparts occurring in the lymph nodes and will not be discussed in this section.

Gastric Marginal –Zone B-cell Lymphoma (Extranodal marginal zone B-cell lymphoma of mucosa-associated lymphatic tissue (MALT) type.)

Synonym: Mucosa associated lymphoid tissue lymphoma (MALT lymphoma)

Definition

This is a primary low grade B-cell lymphoma often associated with H pylori infection occurring most frequently in stomach. It has an indolent behavior and responds well to antibiotic therapy in initial stages. Over the years genetic changes occur and it is transformed to high grade lymphoma. Discrete localized or polypoid tumor, as such, is uncommon and most of these lymphomas are confined to the mucosa and submucosa, and lymph nodal involvement is unusual.

Clinical Findings

The disease is encountered in elderly persons with slight preponderance in males. The patients complain of epigastric pain and dyspepsia, which suggest gastritis or peptic ulcer disease rather than lymphoma. Endoscopic picture shows shallow ulcers, granularity and thickening of mucosal folds suggesting an ill defined infiltrative lesion (61, 62, 63).

The normal gastric mucosa contains sprinkling of lymphocytes and plasma cells but is not known to have organized lymphoid tissue. In the initial stage of primary gastric lymphoma acquisition of organized lymphoid tissue takes place and is usually associated with infection by H Pylori organisms (64). H pylori infection is associated with MALT lymphoma in 62-77% of cases. This association is seen less frequently in high grade lymphoma with a small low grade component and in pure high trade lymphoma of stomach. The organism has been shown to be present in 90% of cases limited to the mucosa and submucosa, falling to 76% when deep submucosa is involved and in 48% of cases with extension beyond the submucosa (65, 66, 67, 68).

Microscopic

Histologically the main finding is the presence of diffuse or vaguely nodular infiltrate of small to medium sized lymphocytes with slightly irregular nuclei and a clear rim of vacuolated cytoplasm, the marginal-zone lymphocytes. In fair number of cases prominent infiltrate of well differentiated plasma cells is seen (Figure 2.1 A-D). The plasma cells often show nuclei with Dutcher bodies and crystalline inclusions. Gastric glands may be disrupted by small clusters of neoplastic cells, giving rise to the so called lymphoepithelial lesion. This finding is quite useful in differentiating inflammatory infiltrate from a lymphomatous lesion. The presence of lymphoid follicles, often with partial replacement by neoplastic cells (follicular colonization), is encountered. The cells in the follicular colonization include monocytoid B cells, some times plasma cells, and not uncommonly large lymphoid cells. The latter cells acquire more genetic abnormality and develop clonal transformation to emerge as a large B cell lymphoma (69, 70 71).

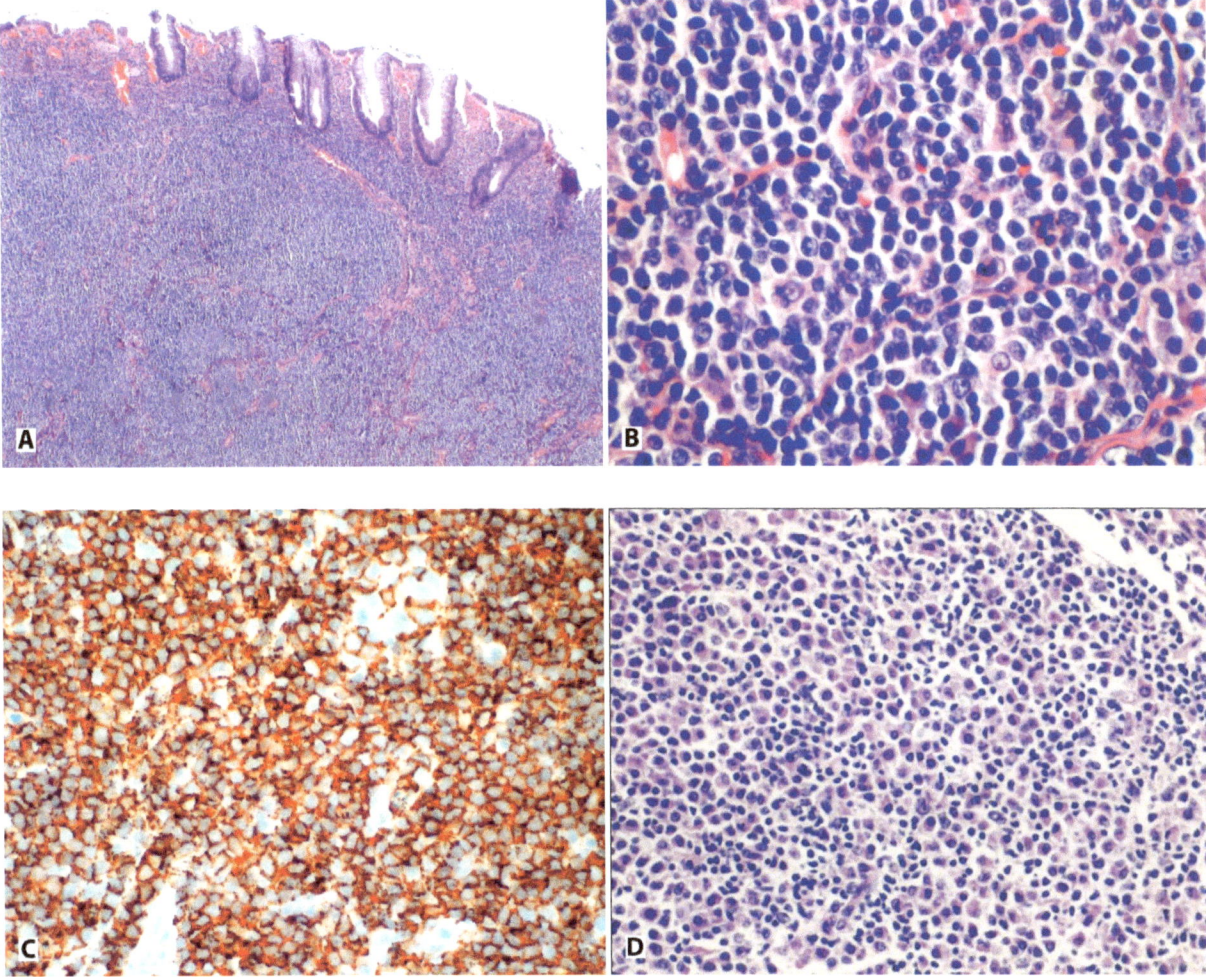

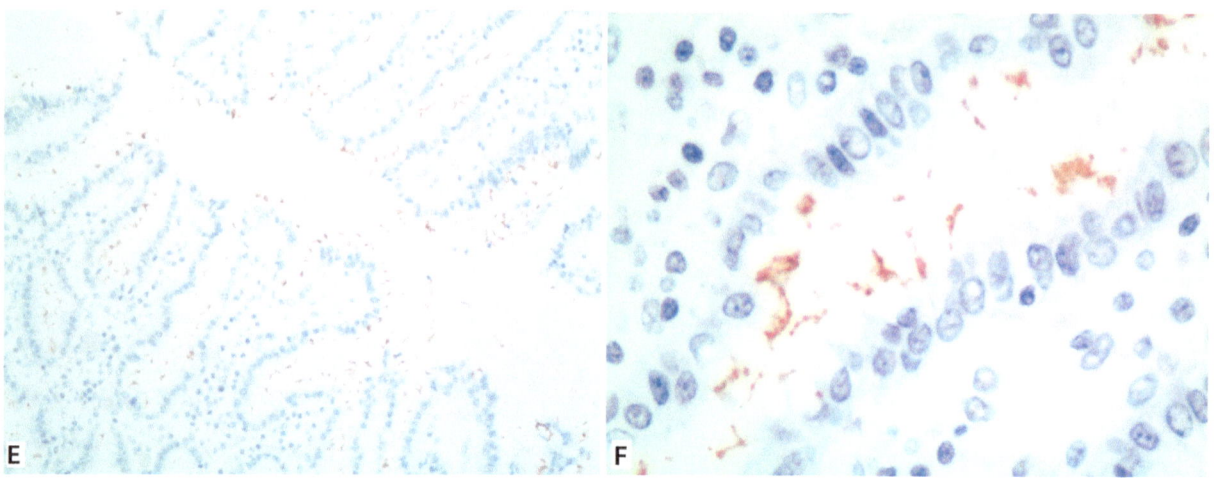

Figure 2.1 Maltoma: (A) a vaguely nodular large lymphocytic infiltrate of lymphocytes in the expanded submucosa, note preservation of surface epithelium and glands (B) the lymphocytes are small to medium sized with oval or slightly irregular nuclei with clear cytoplasm in some (C) all cells express CD 20; (D) the infiltrate in the mucosal lamina propria is rich in plasma cells, which have pink cytoplasm and stand out amidst lymphocytes.(E, F) H Pylori organisms on the surface epithelium and within crevices of crypts (immune stain for H Pylori antigen

Detection of H pylori organisms is fairly easy on routine stains in many cases. However, special stains or immunohistochemical test should be employed in all suspected cases of chronic gastritis and gastric lymphoma. The yield of H pylori will be high in cases of low grade lymphoma, which is located in mucosa and submucosa) in early stage of maltomas. In a series of 399 cases of maltoma, 74.5% cases exhibited complete remission with antibiotic treatment. In these cases, the lymphomatous process is usually restricted to mucosa and submucosa (Figure 2.2A).

Immunophenotyping reveals expression of CD20. Gastric marginal-zone B-cell lymphoma commonly shows translocation t(11;18) (q21;q21) with significant variation in its frequency. This translocation is associated with a high stage disease (Figure 2.2 B) and these patients fail to respond to H pylori antibiotic therapy (72, 73, 74, 75).

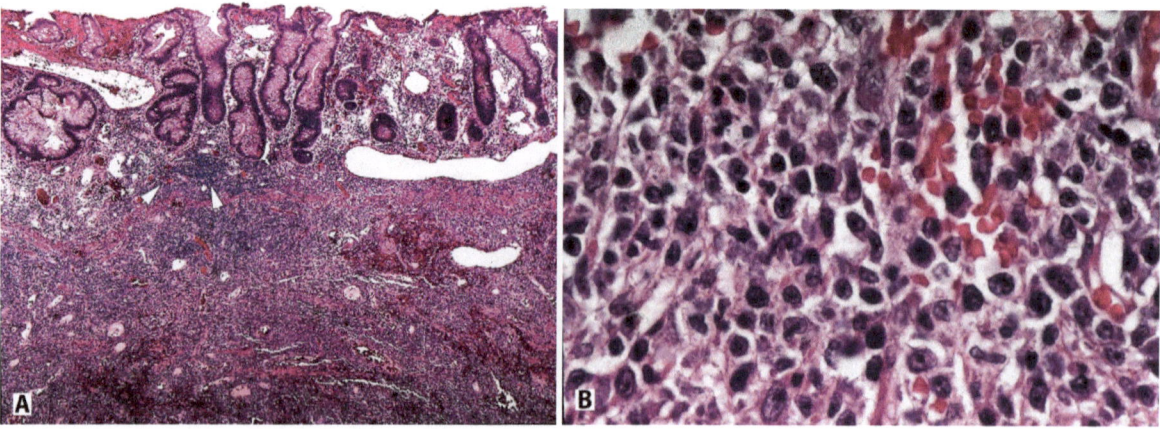

Figure 2.2 (A) small lymphocytic infiltrates in the gastric submucosa (arrow heads) in early phase of maltoma, (B) superimposed diffuse large B cell lymphoma

Evolution of extranodal marginal zone B-cell lymphoma of mucosa-associated lymphatic tissue (MALT) type and Diffuse Large B Cell Lymphoma

These two lymphomas form a spectrum with inflammatory lesion at one end and large B cell lymphoma at the extreme end. An intermediate phase of marked chronic gastritis with features of extranodal marginal-zone B-cell lymphoma is usually present in many cases. On an endoscopic biopsy diagnosis of low grade gastric lymphoma is difficult and careful study of multiple sections from the block is necessary.

The histological features diagnostic of MALToma include B cell clonal proliferation with destructive inflammatory infiltrate and loss of glands, monocytoid B lymphocytes and plasma cells and lymphoepithelial lesions. The extranodal marginal B cell lymphoma (MALToma) should be differentiated from severe chronic gastritis and other low grade B cell lymphoma and incipient diffuse large B cell lymphoma.

Thirty to 65% resistant MALToma are associated with t [11;18] [q21;21] translocation, which is found in 26% of MALToma and 19% of DLBCL (73).

Diffuse large B Cell Lymphoma (DLBCL) of Stomach

This is mainly a disease of older adults and may present with a clinically palpable mass. In its initial stages differentiation from inflammatory lesion is difficult and H pylori bacillary load is high. These cases respond well to antibiotic therapy (Figure 2.2 A) Some cases of DLBCL arise from low grade marginal-zone B-cells by way of large cell transformation of low grade lymphoma (Figure 2.2 B), and all other type of DLBCLs occur de novo (Figure 2.3 A, B). Biopsy at early stage shows monomorphic lymphoid cells, which tend to infiltrate in sheet like manner, and at places sparing the gastric pits and the glands. The cells possess large round or oval irregular or lobated coarse nuclei, distinct nucleoli and narrow but discernible cytoplasm.

Prognosis

In a series of 145 cases of primary B cell gastric lymphoma, 71 cases were of low grade MALTOMA, 25 cases of DLBCL with component of MALTOMA and 49 cases of DLBCL without MALTOMA component. The 5 year survival was 91% for low grade lymphoma, 73% for DLBCL with MALTOMA component and 56% for pure DLBCL. In another such analysis, 92% 5 year survival was found in DLBCL with MALTOMA component , 89% survival in CD 10 +ve DLBCL and 30% survival in CD 10-ve DLBCL (76, 77).

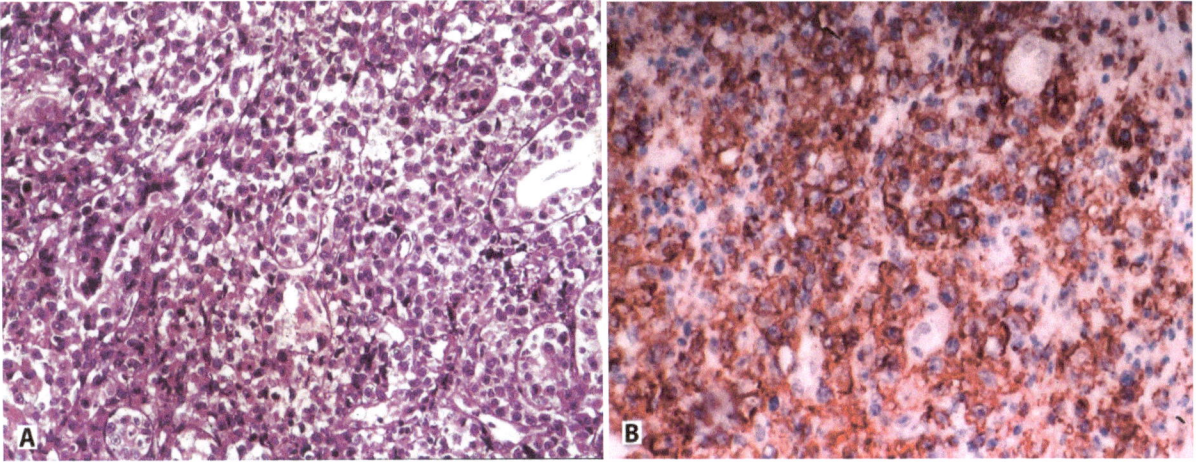

Figure 2.3 (A) Diffuse large B cell lymphoma (de novo) of stomach (B) CD20 prominently expressed in all lymphoma cells (no maltoma component present)

Lymphomas of small intestine

The proportion of malignant lymphoma among all malignant tumors of stomach is low and that for colon is negligible. Whereas, in small intestines, malignant lymphomas account for a good 28% of the total malignant tumors (Table 2.3)

Table 2.3: Malignant Tumors of Small Intestines ($n = 292$) Author's series (1970-2010)	
Adenocarcinoma	126 (43.2%)
Undifferentiated Carcinoma	9 (3.1%)
Metastatic Carcinoma	13 (4.5%)
Lymphoma	**81 (27.7%)**
Leiomyosarcoma	36 (12.3%)
Sarcomas (others + desmoids 3)	9 (3.1%)
Neuroendocrine Tumors	18 (6.2%)

Immunoproliferative Small Intestinal Disease (IPSID)

Synonyms: Mediterranean Lymphoma, Alpha heavy chain disease.

Definition

This is a small intestinal disease characterized by symptoms of malabsorption with associated weight loss and is the result of infiltrate of well differentiated lymphocytes and plasma cells in the mucosa and submucosa. This, in essence, is a low grade lymphoplasmacytic lymphoma and histologically indistinguishable from maltoma rich in plasma cells (see Figure 2.1 D).

Clinical findings

The disease tends to be associated with lower socioeconomic status and most patients are young adults presenting with abdominal pain, malabsorption, diarrhea and weight loss. It has been demonstrated that campylobacter jejuni is an important factor in the genesis of IPSID. Grossly the small bowel may appear normal or show diffuse mural thickening and multiple site involvement in GI tract. Mesenteric lymph nodes are often enlarged. In early phase of IPSID patients respond to broad spectrum antibiotics. The most important laboratory finding is the presence of free alpha heavy chains without associated light chains in the serum of nearly 50% of the patients. The disease in these cases is called alpha heavy chain disease (78, 79, 80, 81, 82).

Microscopic

The small intestinal mucosa shows dense diffuse compact lymphocytic and lymphoplasmacytic infiltrate in the lamina propria, accompanied by much loss of mucosal glands. There is a close similarity of this neoplastic infiltrate with that of marginal zone lymphoma Therefore, IPSID is said to be a special form of maltoma, since immunohistochemically alpha heavy chain deposition can be demonstrated in the lymphoid tissue of IPSID but not in maltoma.

Diffuse Large B cell Lymphoma of Small Intestines (Table 2.7)

Diffuse large B cell lymphoma is usually solitary and ileum is the most commonly affected part followed by jejunum and duodenum. The tumor exhibits a diffusely infiltrating mass with thick rigid hose like appearance (Figure 2.4 A). The overlying mucosa is flattened and ulcerated, but some tumors have a polypoid configuration. Regional lymph nodes are involved in approximately 50% of tumors. Histological features are similar to diffuse large B cell lymphoma occurring anywhere in extra nodal sites or lymph nodes (Figure 2.4 B, C). The lesion is quite aggressive and proportionately long term survival is rather less than malignant lymphoma of stomach and rectum

Diffuse Large B cell Lymphoma of Small Intestines

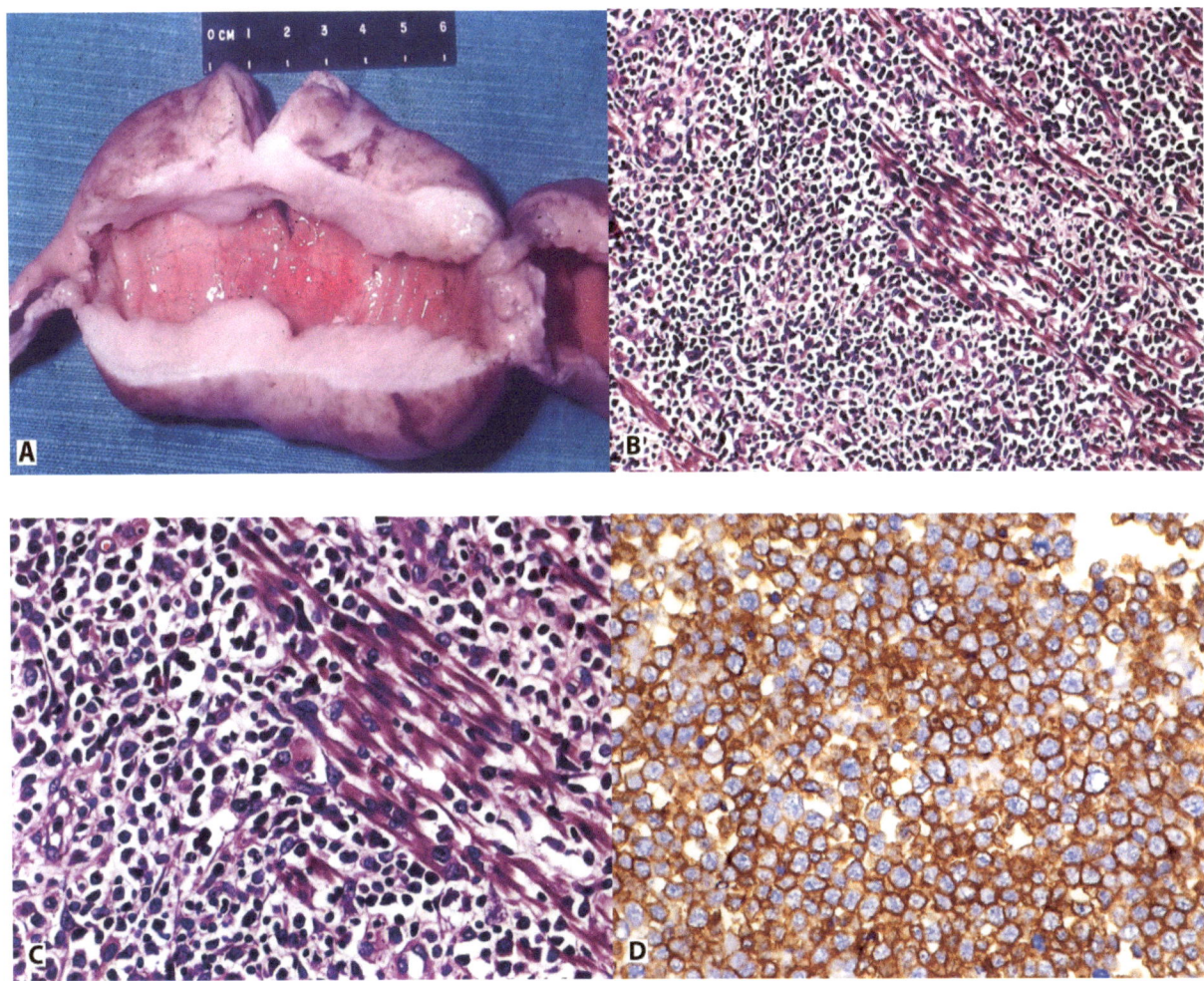

Figure 2.4 Diffuse Large B cell Lymphoma of Small Intestines (A) Homogenous white fleshy solid mass involving loop of small intestine in a circumferential manner (B & C) diffuse large B cell lymphoma infiltrating the wall of small intestines, (D) all lymphoma cells show strong staining for CD 20

Enteropathy-Type Intestinal T-cell Lymphoma

Definition

A peripheral T-cell lymphoma involving small intestine is most often a complication of coeliac disease and histologically characterized by diffuse infiltrate of T-cell lymphocytes in the mucosa and submucosa.

Clinical findings

Over the years, some patients of malabsorption have been shown to develop small intestinal lymphoma. Long term follow up studies of patients with celiac disease reported a 14% incidence of small intestinal lymphoma, which included patients with malabsorption unresponsive to gluten withdrawal and had jejunal ulcers. The patients present with abdominal pain and weight loss and significant number of cases develop acute abdomen due to intestinal perforation.

Microscopic

The lesion appears as a large shallow ulcer with surrounding normal mucosal folds (Figure 2.5 A). No growth, as such, is discernible. Most cases reveal jejunal mucosa infiltrated by sheets of medium to large pleomorphic lymphoid cells (Figure 2.5 B, C), a pattern reminiscent of anaplastic large cell lymphoma. Less commonly the mucosa is replaced by densely packed small monotonous cells. The tumor cells destroy the surface epithelium and superficial parts of crypts leading to shallow ulcers (Figure 2.5A) with histiocytes and particularly eosinophils. A peripheral eosinophilia may also be present. In almost all cases the mucosa away from the neoplastic areas reveals characteristics of coeliac disease. Enteropathy-Type T-cell lymphoma occurs in a subset of cases, who have no history of coeliac disease. However, a subclinical form of coeliac disease may be present and this can be confirmed by demonstration of antibodies to gliadin or HLA phenotype of coeliac disease. Two subtypes of enteropathy-Type intestinal T-cell lymphoma are identified based on CD 56 expression, 21% of lymphomas were CD 56 +ve and with monomorphic population of small to medium lymphoid cells. 79% lymphomas were CD56 –ve and were composed of pleomorphic medium or large cells (Figure 2.5 C, D, E) (83, 84, 85, 86).

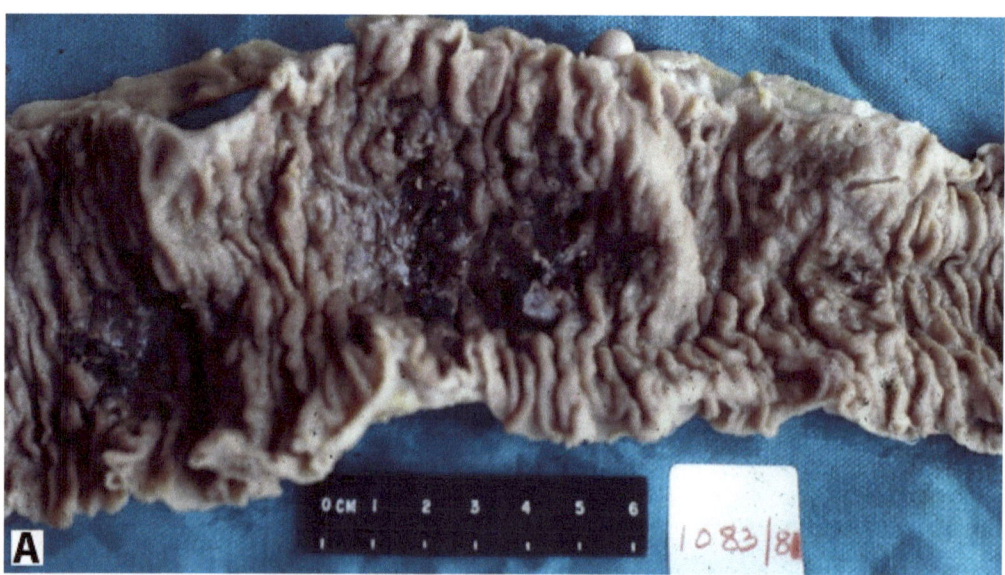

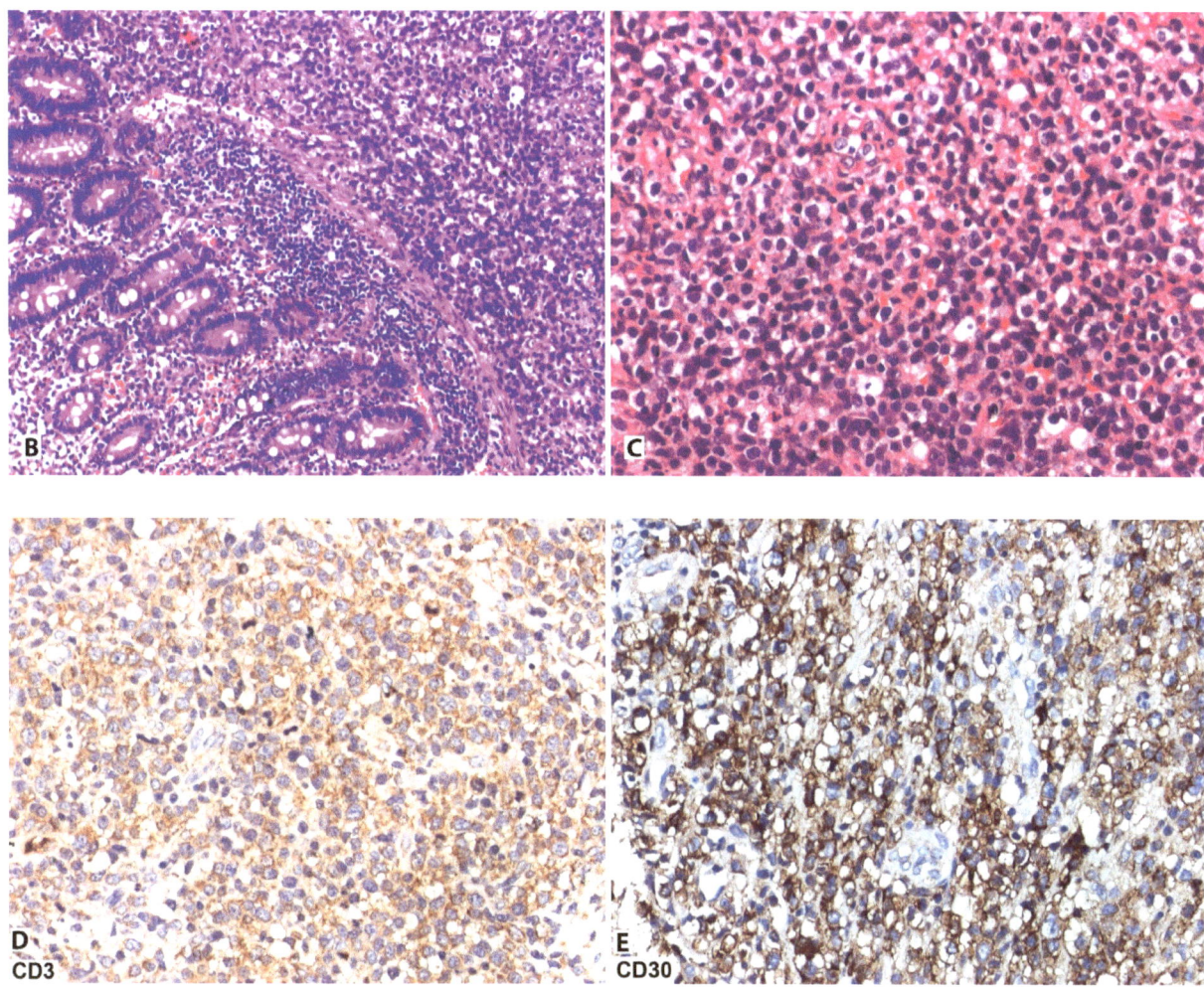

Figure 2.5 Enteropathy-Type Intestinal T-cell Lymphoma (A) Localized ulcerated mucosal lesion of small intestine: (B) marked lymphocytic infiltrate in mucosa and sub mucosa, (C) at higher power large cell pleomorphic lymphoma is evident (D & E) tumor has expressed CD3 prominently and CD30 also stains the lymphomatous cells.

Mantle Cell Lymphoma & Multiple Lymphomatous Polyposis

Definition

This is a unique uncommon clinico-pathological entity characterized by multiple polypoid tumors involving several segments of the gastrointestinal tract, resulting from a lymphomatous involvement of mucosa and submucosa. Majority of cases represent a counter part of mantle cell lymphoma of lymph nodes and the mortality is high.

Clinical Findings

Its prevalence in large series' of gastrointestinal lymphomas is 0.4% (2 of 455 cases of primary GI lymphoma in Japan), 1.7% (2 of 119 lymphomas of small intestines), 5.5% (9 of 165) and 9% (31 of 350 cases of GI lymphoma) (87, 88, 89, 91). The most frequent presenting features are GI bleeding, intestinal obstruction and weight loss. Any portion of GI tract can be involved, and most frequently lymphoma affects multiple sites, particularly ileum, ileo-cecal region and ascending colon. Mesenteric lymph nodes are commonly involved (90, 69). Mantle cell lymphoma generally occurs in adults with a median age of 60 years and male preponderance.

Advanced disease with involvement of regional lymph nodes, liver, spleen or peripheral blood is common at presentation. More than 50% of patients with MCL have bone marrow involvement at the time of diagnosis. Rare cases of multiple lymphomatous polyposis, presenting with multiple intussusceptions, have been reported (92)

Microscopic

A case of mantle Cell Lymphoma presenting as a large single colonic mass: vaguely nodular infiltrate of atypical lymphoid cells with partly preserved mucosa is present. Remnants of reactive lymphoid follicles may be seen (Figure 2.6 A, B, C). The infiltrate tends to displace and obliterate the mucosal glands but lymphoepithelial lesions are rare. This case did not have multiple polyposis.

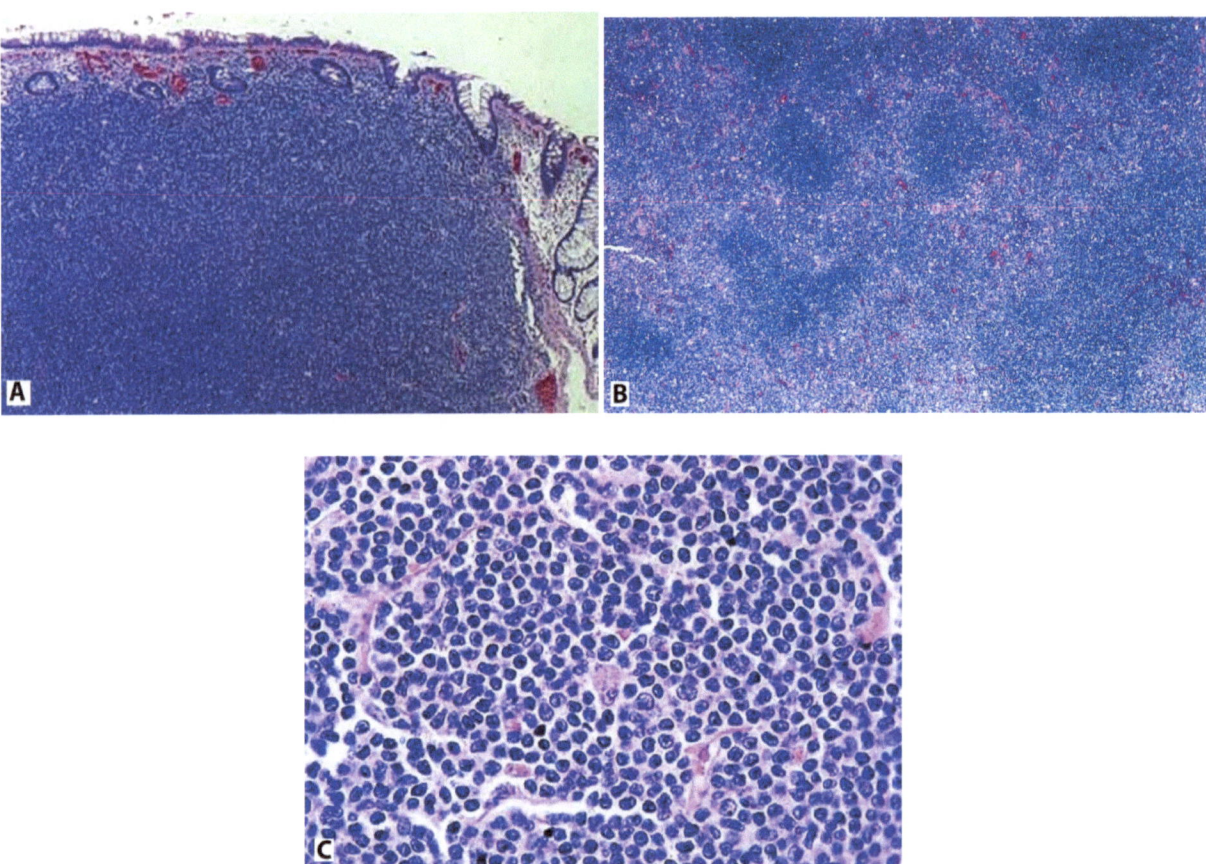

Figure 2.6 Mantle cell lymphoma (A) lymphoma involving the wall of colon with reasonably intact mucosal glands, note vague nodular pattern ((B) Remnants of lymphoid follicles seen (C) atypical lymphoid cells, slightly larger and more irregular than normal lymphocytes

A case of multiple lymphomatous polyposis (mantle cell type)

Diagnostic immunophenotype includes expression of cyclin D1, CD20, CD5 and CD 79a; CD 23 and CD 10 are not expressed. (Figure 2.7 A, B, C, D, E, F) (68, 93)

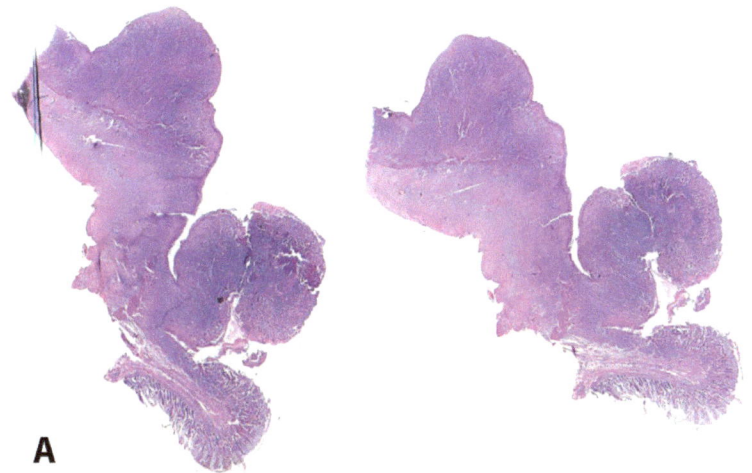
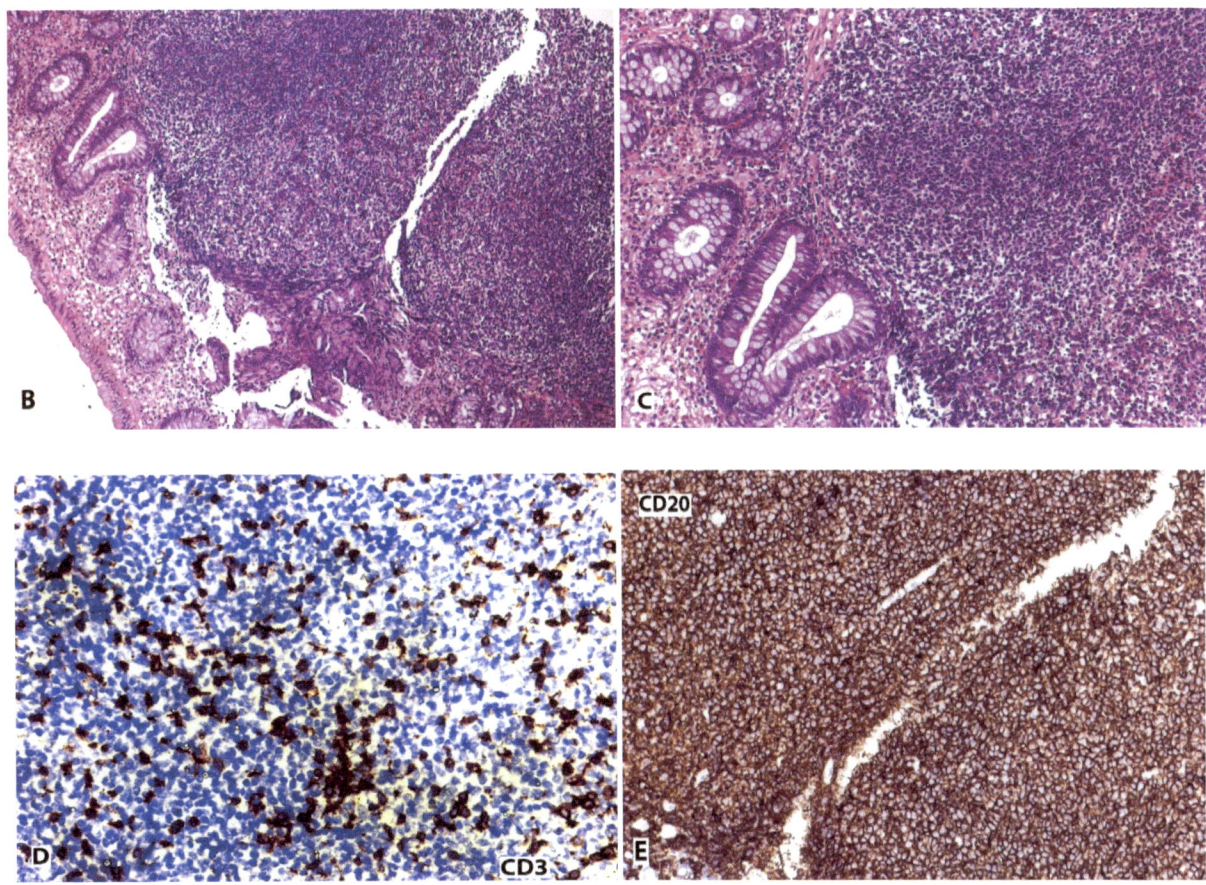

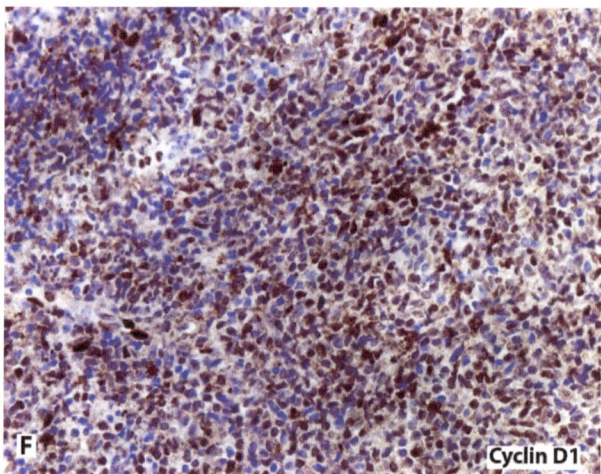

Figure 2.7 Another case of lymphomatous polyposis: (A) three small polypoid projections seen (B & C) nodular architecture of this colonic lymphoma, note preservation of superficial mucosa and surface epithelium, (D) CD3 expressed by few reactive T lymphocytes), (E) lymphoma cells are CD20 positive (F) tumor cells strongly express Cyclin D1 in the nuclei (Courtesy Dr Sushmita Dave, pathologist. Rajkot (Gujarat)

Differential Diagnosis

There are some instances of lymphomas other than mantle cell type which display endoscopic and gross appearance of lymphomatous polyposis. Follicular lymphoma, marginal zone lymphoma immunoproliferative small intestinal disease (EPSID), enteropathy-associated T-cell lymphoma and nodular lymphoid hyperplasia have shown endoscopic appearance of lymphomatous polyposis (94, 95, 96, 97, 98). A careful histological and immunohistochemical study is necessary to distinguish these conditions from mantle cell lymphoma, which has a rather poor prognosis. Cyclin D1 positive immunostain is pathognomonic of mantle cell lymphoma (Figure 2.7F).

References for extranodal lymphoma

59 Koch P, del Valle F, Berdel W, et al: Primary gastrointestinal non-Hodgkin's lymphoma: 1. Anatomic and histologic distribution, clinical features and survival data of 371 patients registered in the German multicenter study GIT NHL 01/92. J Clin Oncol 2001; 19:3861-3873

60 Ghimire P, Wu GY, Zhu L: Primary gastrointestinal lymphoma. World J Gastroenterol 2011; 17: 697-707

61 Hatano B, Ohshima K, Tsuchiya T et, el: Clinicopathological features of gastric B-cell lymphoma: A series of 317 cases. Pathol Int 2002; 5t2: 677-682

62 Zucca E, Bertoni F, Roggero E, et, el: The gastric marginal zone B-cell lymphoma of MALT type. Blood 2000; 96: 410-419

63 Yokoi T, Nakamura T, Kasugai K, et , al: primary low-grade gastric mucosa-associated lymphoid tissue (MALT) lymphoma with polypoid appearance: Polypoid gastric MALT lymphoma-A clinicopathological study of eight cases. Pathol Int 1999; 49:702-709

64 Genta RM, Hammer HW, Graham DY: Gastric lymphoid follicles in Helicobacter pylori infection: frequency, distribution, and response to triple therapy. Human Pathol. 1993; 24: 577-583.

65 Karat D, O'Hanion DM, Hayes N, st al: prospective study of H pylori infection in primary gastric lymphoma. Br J Surg 1995; 82:1369-1370

66 Gisbertz IA, Jonkers DM, Aronds GM, et al: Specific detection of H Pylori and non-H pylori flora in small- and large- cell primary gastric B cell lymphoma. Ann Oncol 1997; 8 Suppl 2: 33-36

67 Bouzourene H, Haefliger T, Delacretaz F, Saraga E: The role of H pylori in primary gastric MALT lymphoma. Histopathology 1999; 34: 18-23.

68 Nakamura S, Yao T, Aoyagi K, et al: H pylori and primary gastric lymphoma. A histopathologic and immunohistochemical analysis of 237 patients Cancer 1997; 79: 3-11.

69 Isaacson PG: Gastrointestinal lymphoma. Human Pathol 1994; 25: 1020-1029

70 Chan J: Gastrointestinal lymphomas: an overview with emphasis on new findings and diagnostic problems. Semin Diag Pathol 1996; 13: 260-296.

71 Isaacson PG, Wotherspoon AC, Diss T pan Lx. Follicular colonization in B cell lymphoma of mucosa-associated lymphoid tissue. Am J Surg Pathol 1991; 15: 819-828

72 Dierlamm J, Baens M, Stefanove-Quzounova, et, al: Detection of t(11;18) (q21;q21) by interphase fluorescence in situ hybridization using AP12 and MLT specific probes. Blood 2000; 96: 2215-2218

73 Liu H, Ruskone-Foumestraux A, Lavaergne-Slove A, et , al: Resistance of t(11;18) positive gastric mucosa-associated lymphoid tissue lymphoma to Helicobacter pylori eradication therapy. Lancet 2001; 357: 39-40

74 Ye H, Liu H, Raderer M, et al: High incidence of t(11;18) (q21; q21}in Helicobacter pylori-negative gastric MALT lymphoma. Blood 2003; 101: 2547-2550

75 Isaacson PG: Gastrointestinal lymphomas of T- and B-cell type. Mod Pathol 1999; 12: 151-158

76 Cogliatti SB, Schmid U, Schumacher U, et al: Primary B cell gastric lymphoma: a clinicopathological study of 145 patients. Gastroenterology 1991; 101: 1159-1170

77 Takeshita M, Iwashsita A, Kurihara K, et al: Histologic and immunohistologic findings and prognosis of 40 cases of gastric large B-cell lymphoma. Am J Surg Pathol 2000:;24: 1641-1649

78 Al-Saleem T, Al-Mondhiry H: Immunoproliferative small intestinal disease (IPSID) A model for mature B-cell neoplasms Blood 2005; 105: 2274-2280

79 Tabbane F, Mourali N, Cammoun M, et al: Results of laparotomy in immunoproliferative small intestinal disease. Cancer 1988; 61: 1699-1706

80 Lecuit M: Immunoproliferative small intestinal disease associated with Campylobacter jejuni. J Natl Cancer Inst 2004; 96: 571-573

81 Lecuit M, Abachin E, Martin A, et al: Immunoproliferative small intestinal disease associated with Campylobacter jejuni. N Engl J Med 2004; 350: 239-248

82 Fine K, Stone M: Alpha-heavy chain disease, Mediterranean lymphoma, and immunoproliferative small intestinal disease. Am J Gastroenterol 1999; 94: 1139-1152

83 Isaacson PG: Relation between cryptic intestinal lymphoma and refractory sprue. Lancer 2000; 356: 178-79

84 Chott A, Vesely M, Simonitsch I, et al: Classification of intestinal T-cell neoplasms and their differential diagnsis. Am J Clin Pathol 1999; 111: S68-74

85 Gale J, Simmonds P, Mead G, et al; Enteropathy-Type Intestinal T-cell lymphoma: Clinical features and treatment of 31 patients in a single center J Clin Pathol 2000; 18: 795-803

86 Chott A, Haedickle W, Mosberger I, et al: Most CD 56+ Intestinal lymphomas are CD8+, CD5- T-cell lymphomas of monomorphic small to medium size histology. Am J Pathol 1998; 153:1483-1490

87 Domizio P, Owen RA, Shepherd NA, et al: Primary Lymphoma of the Small Intestine: A clinicopathological study of 119 cases. Am J Surg Pathol 1993; 17:429-442

88 Ruskone Fourmestraux A Delmer A, Lavergne A. Multiple lymphomatous polyposis of the gastrointestinal tract: a prospective clinico-pathologic study of 31 cases. Gastroenterology 1997;112: 7-18

89 Moynihan MJ, Bast MA, Chan WC, et al: Lymphomatous polyposis: A neoplasm of either follicular mantle or germinal center cell origin. Am J Surg Pathol 1996; 20:442-452.

90 Kiodoma T, Ohshima K, Nomura K, et al: Lymphomatous polyposis of gastrointestinal tract, including mantle cell lymphoma, follicular lymphoma and mucosa-associated lymphoid tissue lymphoma. Histopathology 2005; 47: 467-478

91 Nakamura S, Matsumoto T, Mitsuo L, et al: Primary gastrointestinal lymphoma in Japan: A clinicopathological Analysis of 455 patients with Special Reference to Its Time Trend. Cancer 2003; 97: 2462-2473

92 Kella VKN, Constantine R, Parikh NS, et al: Mantle cell lymphoma of the gastrointestinal tract presenting with multiple intussusceptions-case report and review of literature. World Journal of Surgical Oncology 2009; 7: 60-65

93 O'Briain DS, Kennedy MJ, Daly PA, et al: Multiple lymphomatous polyposis of the gastrointestinal tract. A clinicopathologically distinctive form of non-Hodgkin's lymphoma of B-cell centrocytic type Am J Surg Pathol 1989; 13: 691-699

94 LeBrun DP, Kamel OW, Cleary ML, et al: Follicular lymphomas of the Gastrointestinal Tract: Pathologic features in 31 cases and bcl-2 Oncogenic Protein Expression Am J Pathol 1992; 140: 1327-1335

95 Kodoma T, Ohshima K, Nomura K, et al: Lymphomatous polyposis of of the gastrointestinal tract, including mantle cell lymphoma, follicular lymphoma and mucosa-associated lymphoid tissue lymphoma. Histopathology 2005; 47: 467-478

96 Ramot B, Shahin N, Dbis J: Malabsorption syndrome in lymphoma of small intestine. A study of 13 cases. Isr J Med Sci 1965; 1: 221-226

97 Hirakawa K, Fuchigami T, Nakamura S, et al: Primary Gastrointestinal T-cell Lymphoma resembling multiple lymphomatous polyposis. Gastroenterology 1996; 111: 778-782

98 Ranchod M, Lewin K, Dorfman R. Lymphoid hyperplasia of the gastrointestinal tract. A study of 26 cases and review of literature. Am J Surg Pathol 1978; 2: 383-400

Gastro-Entero-Pancreatic Endocrine Tumors

The Dispersed Neuroendocrine System

Introduction

Oberndorfer in 1907 described special tumors of the small intestines, which he called "Karzinoide Tumoren" [carcinoids] 99. Little did he realize that his discovery will lead to an uncharted territory, the 'dispersed neuroendocrine system'. The journey from carcinoid to neuroendocrine system has been fascinating, tortuous, long, and spanning a period of nearly 100 years after the seminal contribution of Oberndorfer. The nervous system comprises the conventional somatic and autonomic divisions and now includes the neuroendocrine system. The neuroendocrine cells occur in pituitary, adrenal medulla, thyroid [C cell], parathyroid, paraganglia, broncho-pulmonary and gastrointestinal endocrine cells, pancreatic islets, Merkel cell of skin and miscellaneous sites such as breast, cervix, prostate, larynx etc. And some of the unusual primary sites include kidney, paranasal sinuses, liver, gall bladder, middle ear, eye, orbit and mesentery. (99)

Origin of Neuroendocrine Cells

Feyrter [1938] suggested that the GI endocrine cells formed an integral part of a diffuse endocrine system, in which constituent cells are diffusely scattered in singles or small groups throughout the tissues of the body. He believed that the endocrine cells arose from the mucosa of the gut and is, therefore, derived from the endoderm (100). Pearse [1969] described the cytochemical characteristics of the cells of the dispersed neuroendocrine system [DNS] and coined the acronym 'APUD' [Amine Precursor Uptake Decarboxylase]. He propounded that the cells, to be called neuroendocrine cells, arose from the neural crest and migrated to various sites in alimentary and respiratory systems, and conventional endocrine organs.(101)

The subject of embryological derivation of neuroendocrine cells of the gastrointestinal and respiratory system is controversial but now it is accepted that the endocrine cells of gastrointestinal tract and pancreas are derived from specialized cells in the embryonic GI system (endoderm), which can differentiate into endocrine and acinar cells. The neural crest origin of cells of the anterior pituitary, thyroidal C cells, chromaffin cells of adrenal medulla and certain cells of paragangliomas is well accepted. It is futile to ponder over the exact embryological origin of neuroendocrine cell. Instead, we should focus on the amalgamation of the neural and endocrine physiologic mechanisms which are integral to the neuroendocrine system (102).

Definition of Neuroendocrine cells

These are cells that receive neuronal input [transmitters released by nerve cells] and, as a consequence of this input, release message molecules [hormones] to the blood. In this way they bring about integration between nervous system and the endocrine system, a process known as neuroendocrine integration.

Identification of Neuroendocrine Cells

All neuroendocrine cells are readily identified by immunohistochemical staining for neuron-specific enolase [NSE], chromogranin and synaptophysin. In all suspected cases of neuroendocrine tumors, these stains are regularly employed and found to be consistently positive and reliable. Electron microscopy invariably shows dense core neurosecretory granules measuring from 150 to 400 nm in size in all neuroendocrine cells and their lesions.

Nomenclature

Neuroendocrine cells and their tumors are subdivided into hormonally functioning and non-functioning types. The hormone secreting neuroendocrine tumors are labeled according to the type of the hormone secreted or presenting clinical syndromes (for example insulinoma, see Table 3.1)

Enterochromaffin (EC) cells (Kulchitsky cells) are a type of enteroendocrine cells occurring in the epithelial lining of the digestive tract and the respiratory tract and contain about 90% of the body's store of serotonin (5-Hydroxy tryptamine). The cells are stimulated by gastrin molecule that is produced in the antrum of the stomach by G cells.

The other population of chromaffin cells found only in the stomach is called enterochromaffin-like cells (ECL). They look like EC cells but do not contain 5-HT. ECL cells respond to gastrin released by G-cells and release histamine which stimulates parietal cells to secrete gastric acid.

Anatomical Distribution and Functions of Cells of Neuroendocrine System

Hormones of gastro-entero-pancreatic endocrine system are all peptides and as of 1925 three peptides, namely secretin, gastrin and cholecystokinin [CCK] were described. The list of peptides has grown exponentially to over 30 peptides in the last 5 decades. The anatomical location and functions of various cells are tabulated below.

Table 3.1: Established Peptide Hormones

	Distribution	Functions
Cholecystokinin diminishing towards ileum	Numerous in duodenum, moderate in jejunum	stimulates contraction of gall bladder and pancreatic secretions
Secretin	Concentration highest in duodenum followed by Jejunum	stimulates pancreatic bicarbonate secretion and counteracts duodenal acidification
Gastric Inhibitory Peptide [GIP]	Duodenum and jejunum	inhibits secretion of gastric acid enhances insulin secretions
Enkephalin	Found through out the gut Particularly in antrum & upper duodenum	increases muscle tone & gastric emptying, controls pain
Motilin	Widely distributed in GI tract from esophagus To anus, also gall bladder and biliary tract	controls activity of gastrointestinal musculature
Substance P	Through out GI tract with highest in small bowel, Also in central & peripheral nervous systems	stimulates intestinal peristalsis; modulates esophageal sphincter & gall bladder contraction

Table 3.2: Peptide Hormones Associated with Syndromes	Distribution	Functions
Gastrin [G cells]	Largest population found in gastric antrum Duodenum major source of extra-antral Gastrin	Major action: stimulation of HCL secretions from parietal cells; also stimulates pepsin and intrinsic factor
Glucagon [A cells]	Exclusively in alpha cells of islets Of Langerhans Glucagon imunoreactivity found in certain Intestinal and neural cells but do not secrete Glucagon	Glycogenolysis and gluconeogenesis in liver
Insulin [B cells]	Exclusively secreted by beta cells of islets Of Langerhans	Increases glucose intake & utilization, increases lipogenesis, general anabolic Effect
Pancreatic Polypeptides [PP]	Cells in periphery of islets of head of pancreas & dispersed in exocrine Pancreas	Suppression of exocrine pancreatic secretions & gall bladder contractions
Somatostatin {D Cell}	Found throughout the central nervous, gastrointestinal and genitourinary systems Also found in thyroid, adrenal medulla thymus, spleen & salivary glands, highest. Concentration in duodenum & pancreas, also In myenteric plexuses and mucosa of GI tract	Widespread inhibitory actions on GI tract pituitary and pancreatic peptides; inhibits release of gastrin, secretin, CCK, GIP Motilin, VIP, insulin, glucagon, pancreatic PP, growth hormone & TSH
Vasoactive Intestinal Peptide [VIP]	Concentrated mainly in GI tract with large amounts in the nerves of intestinal wall; also Found in brain and genitourinary tract	Most important function is vasodilatation, smooth muscle contraction and secretions of intestinal and genitourinary tracts

Neuroendocrine tumors of gastrointestinal tract and pancreas

General Considerations (Tables 3.3, 3.4)

The term carcinoid is well entrenched in the medical literature and is synonymous with the term neuroendocrine tumor. The term APUDOMA, which also means carcinoid/neuroendocrine tumor, is now abandoned. WHO 2000 on neuroendocrine classification retained the term carcinoid but, 2003 WHO classification has replaced this term with endocrine tumor/endocrine carcinoma.

The tumors arising from neuroendocrine cells are all identical morphologically, regardless of the anatomical site and whether functional or nonfunctional. The functioning tumor is identified on the basis of clinical presentation and determination of hormone level in blood by RIA.

Table 3.3: Classification of Gastro-entero-pancreatic Endocrine Tumors [103]

Stomach	Cell of origin	Main hormone produced
Carcinoid tumor type I	ECL	Histamine
Carcinoid tumor type II	ECL	Histamine
Carcinoid tumor type III	ECL	Histamine
Gastrinoma	G	Gastrin
Duodenum		
Gastrinoma	G	Gastrin
Somatostatinoma	D	Somatostatin
Gangliocytic paraganglioma	?	Somatostatin, PP
Carcinoid tumor	EC	Serotonin
Small intestine & cecum		
Carcinoid tumor	EC	Serotonin
Rectum & sigmoid colon		
Carcinoid tumor	EC	Serotonin
Pancreas		
Insulinoma	B cell	Insulin
Gastrinoma	G cell	Gastrin
Glucagonoma	A cell	Glucagon
VIPoma	not known	Vasoactive intestinal peptide
Somatostatinoma	D cell	Somatostatin, ACTH, Calcitonin etc

(Kloppel G, Perren A, Heitz PU: The Gastroenteropancreatic Neuroendocrine Cell System and Its Tumors: The WHO classification. Ann. N. Y. Acad. Sci 2004; 1014:13-27)[103]

Table 3.4: Grading of Gastro-entero-pancreatic endocrine tumors [103]

(A) Well differentiated endocrine tumor	
Grade I (Benign behavior)	Non-functioning, histologically bland, <1 cm Mucosa-submucosa, non-angioinvasive
Grade II (malignancy uncertain)	Non-functioning, histologically bland, 1-2 cm Mucosa-submucosa, sometimes angioinvasive
(B) Well differentiated endocrine carcinoma	
Grade III (low grade malignant)	Sometimes functional, bland, >2 cm, extension beyond submucosa, with or without angioinvasion
(C) Poorly differentiated endocrine carcinoma	
Grade IV (high grade malignant)	Cytologically poorly differentiated, some functioning others not functioning, poor prognosis

(Kloppel G, Perren A, Heitz PU: The Gastroenteropancreatic Neuroendocrine Cell System and Its Tumors: The WHO classification. Ann. N. Y. Acad. Sci 2004; 1014:13-27)103

Prevalence of Neuroendocrine tumors of digestive system

Modlin et al presented a 5-decade analysis of 13,715 carcinoid tumors, which represents the largest epidemiology series addressing carcinoid tumors from various sites in the body (Table 3.5)104.

Table 3.5 Prevalence of carcinoid tumors [104]

Site	No of Cases
Small intestine	3938 (41.8%)
Rectum	2581 (27.4%)
Appendix	1679 (17.8%)

(Adapted from Modlin IM, Lye KD, Kidd M: A 5-decade Analysis of 13,715 Carcinoid Tumors. Cancer 2003; 97: 934-959 104

Neuroendocrine Tumors (NET) of Stomach

Definition

The majority of endocrine tumors of the stomach are well differentiated, non-functioning enterochromaffin-like (ECL) cell carcinoids arising from oxyntic mucosa of the gastric body and fundus.

Clinical Findings

Neuroendocrine tumors of the stomach arise from enterochromaffin like cells (ECL), and NETs from all other sites in GI tract arise from enterochromaffin cells (EC). ECL cells secrete histamine, while EC cells secrete serotonin. EC cell carcinoid is extremely rare in stomach and hence gastric carcinoid tumors do not give rise to

Carcinoid Syndrome. On the basis of pathophysiology, three types of ECL cell gastric carcinoids are identified 105, 106:

Type 1) Autoimmune chronic atrophic gastric or treatment with proton pump inhibitors, which destroy parietal cells giving rise to achlorhydria and hypergastrinemia (Diagram 1)

Type 2) Associated with multiple endocrine neoplasia (MEN 1) and Zollinger-Ellison syndrome with associated gastrinoma producing hypergastrinemia (Diagram 1)

Type 3) Occurring sporadically (spontaneous) and not associated with hypergastrinemia.

Microscopic

It is necessary to know the various cell types normally occurring in gastric glands of fundus and body of stomach (Table 3.6) in order to understand the pathogenesis of ECL cell carcinoid and its surrounding milieu.

Table 3.6: Cells of Gastric Glands and Secretory products	
Chief cell	Pepsinogen
Parietal cell	Acid, Intrinsic factor
Endocrine Cells	
G cells (mainly antral)	Gastrin
D cells (sparse & central)	Somatostatin
ECL cell	Histamine (Fundus & body)

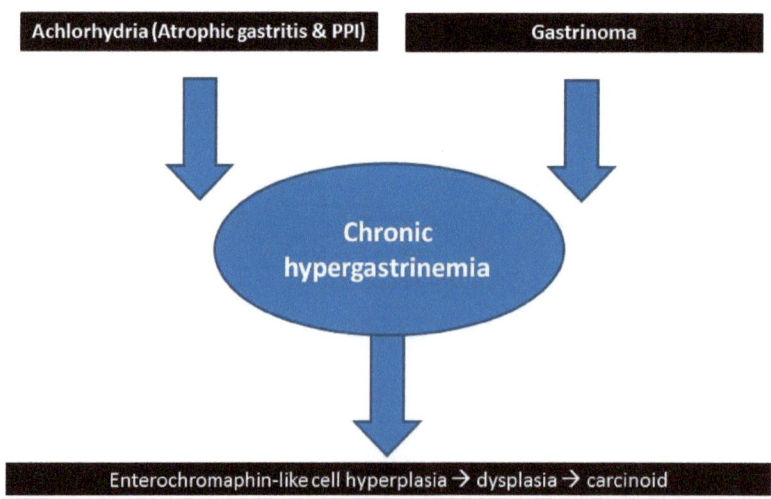

Diagram 1: modified and adopted from, Bordi C, D'Adda T, Azzoni C, Ferraro G: Pathogenesis of ECL tumors in humans. Yale J Biol Med. 2003; 71: 273-284 107

Type 1 gastric carcinoids

In autoimmune gastritis, circulating auto antibodies cause selective destruction of acid secreting parietal cells, which lead to a state of hypergastrinemia. This also occurs in proton pump inhibitor drugs used in cases for therapeutic reduction of gastric acid and in cases of H pylori induced severe chronic gastritis. Hypergastrinemia will give rise to small nodules of ECL cell hyperplasia, which may lead to dysplasia and eventually carcinoid tumor. Type 1 carcinoids appear as tan nodules or polyps within the mucosa, majority <1 cm, and are multiple in 57% of cases (Figure. 3.1). Bulk of Type 1 gastric carcinoids behave in an entirely benign fashion, a few will invade the muscularis propria (Figure 1B, IC). (108,109,110,111,112)

Type 2 gastric carcinoids (Zollinger Ellison Syndrome)

These arise from ECL cells in the body mucosa in a background of ECL cell hyperplasia secondary to a gastrin producing carcinoid in the duodenum or pancreas. About 20% of cases of ZES are associated with MEN 1 syndrome. The risk of development of Type 2 carcinoid is almost 100 times greater in MEN 1 associated ZES than in sporadic ZES. The mortality for Type 2 is largely dependent on the stage of associated gastrinoma but is about 10%

Type 3 gastric carcinoids of EC cells

They are rather uncommon in stomach and are often bulky tumors with local lymph node metastases at presentation. Transmural invasion and serosal involvement are commonly seen. This tumor is akin to small cell undifferentiated or "oat" cell bronchogenic carcinoma in its structure and behavior. The mortality rate for Type 3 carcinoid is in the range of 25%-30%

A particularly aggressive gastric neuroendocrine tumor has been described. These are heterogeneous with multidirectional differentiation - combined glandular and endocrine components. Transmural invasion, serosal infiltration and metastasis to regional lymph nodes are often seen at the time of presentation.112, 113

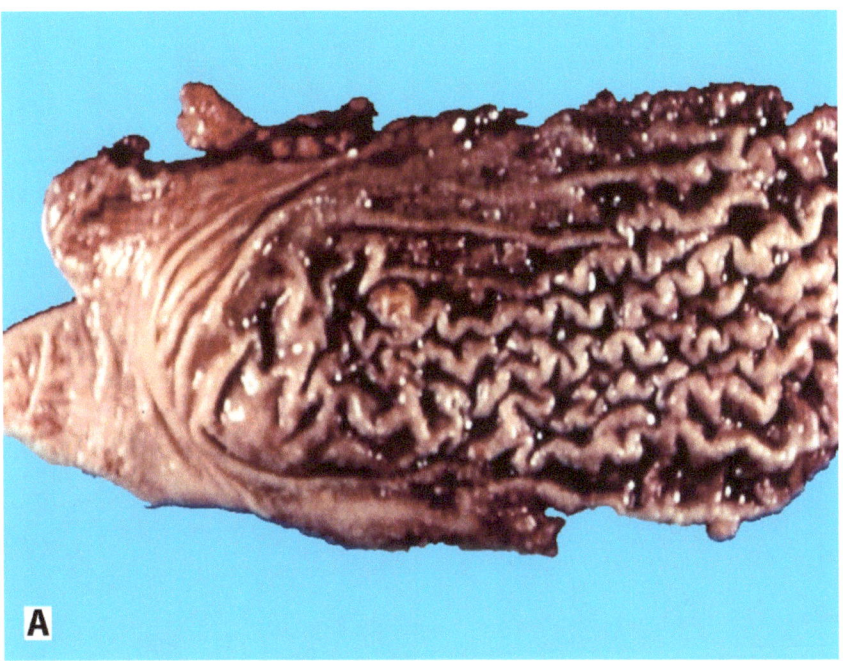

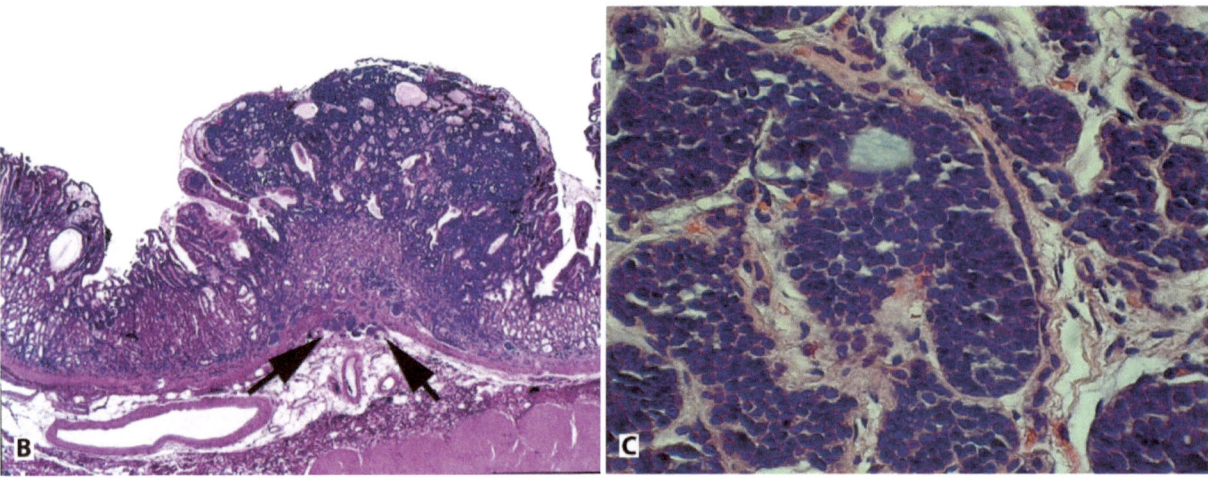

Figure. 3.1 Multiple neuroendocrine tumors: (A) multiple small nodules of carcinoid tumor over mucosa of resected stomach (B) one of the tumors of stomach showing infiltration in submucosa (arrows) (C) high magnification of small round cells arranged in solid nests separated by delicate stroma

Carcinoid tumors (NETs) of small intestine (including duodenum)

(Figure. 3.2)

Definition

Endocrine tumors of small intestine reveal differences according to the anatomical site and type specific endocrine cells involved in tumor formation (Table 3.3): classification of gastroenteropancreatic tumors: (103)

The basic morphology and grading will be similar or common to all types of functioning or non- functioning neuroendocrine tumors of duodenum, jejunum and ileum Table 3.4 (103).

Duodenal Neuroendocrine Tumors

These include gastrinoma, somatostatinoma, serotonin secreting tumor, VIPoma and Gangliocytic paraganglioma.

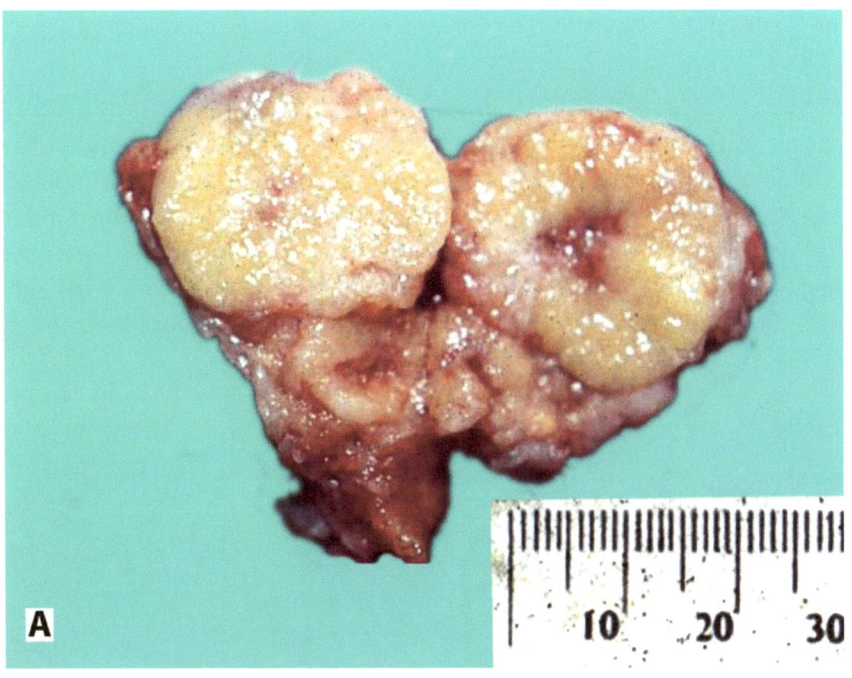

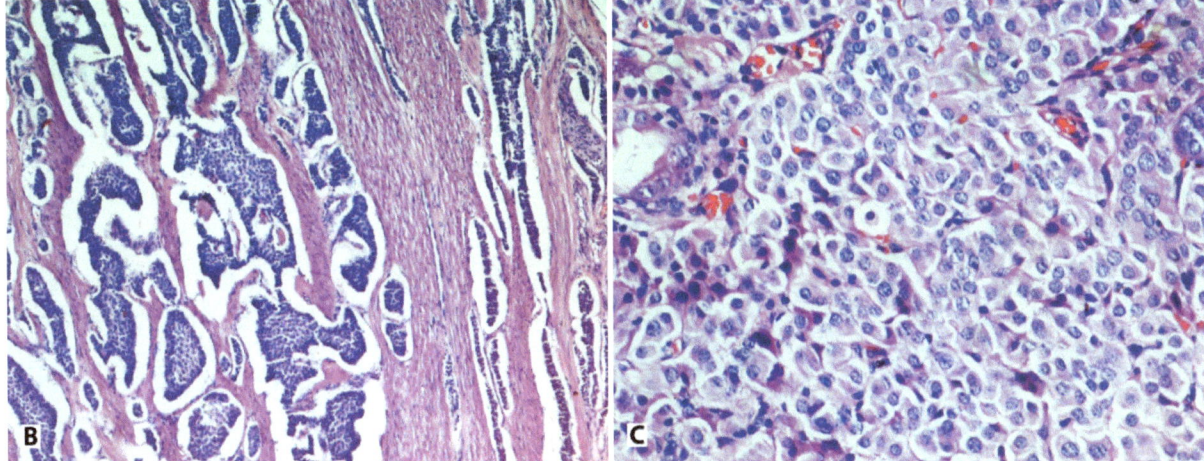

Figure 3.2 Carcinoid tumor of duodenum (non-functioning): (A) a 2 cm yellowish white nodule occupying submucosa and muscularis (B) islands of small cells infiltrating deep into muscularis (C) sheets of neuroendocrine cells containing round pale staining nuclei with fine chromatin

Clinical findings:

The presenting features include bleeding, polypoid mucosal growth, excess hormone induced symptoms [gastrinoma, Somatostatinoma, carcinoid syndrome], jaundice (ampullary tumors) and in few cases symptoms of associated neurofibromatosis (NF 1).

Gastrin-Producing (G cell) neuroendocrine tumors (Gastrinoma)

This is the most frequent subtype of duodenal NET, accounting for over 60% of NETs at this site. About 30% exhibit lymph node metastasis. Generally all hormone secreting endocrine tumors are mostly low grade malignant tumors. Gastrinoma, not infrequently, is encountered in a syndrome of multiple endocrine neoplasia (MEN 1) (110, 114). The subject of gastrinoma is further described in detail in the section on pancreatic neuroendocrine tumors (NETs)

Somatostatin-Producing (D cell) NET

This lesion is characterized by its frequent occurrence in periampullary region, association with von Recklinghausen syndrome in 30% of cases, and presence of pseudo acini with psammoma bodies histologically (Figure. 3.3). It has been commonly misdiagnosed as adenocarcinoma. The symptoms induced by somatostatin hormone are not dramatic or readily diagnostic. The patients display moderate hyperglycemia, cholelithiasis and constipation. Dayal and others compared duodenal carcinoids from patient with and without associated neurofibromatosis and found that 8 of 9 carcinoids with associated VR disease were pure somatostatinomas. (115, 116)

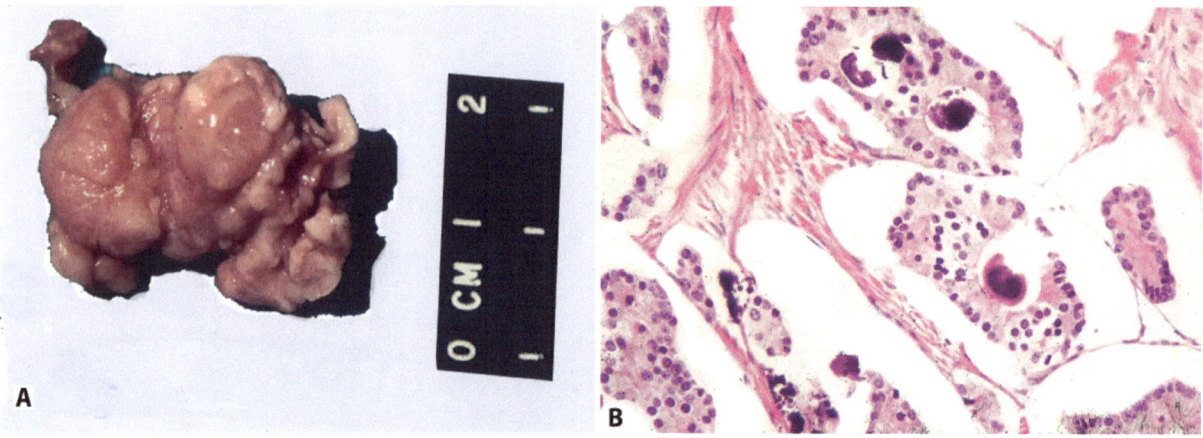

Figure. 3.3 (A) nodule < 1cm in periampullary pancreatic tissue (B) presence of pseudoacini with psammoma bodies can be mistaken as adenocarcinoma

Serotonin-Producing NET

This is the classical carcinoid tumor characterized by no known predisposing condition, nested growth pattern and serotonin secretions. It may metastasize to liver and give rise to typical carcinoid syndrome. (116, 117)

Gangliocytic Paraganglioma

(Figure. 3.4 A-G)

This unique neuroendocrine tumor arises almost exclusively in the II part of the duodenum and particularly in ampullary region. The lesion is typically submucosal, nodular, polypoid, 2-4 cm in size and may cause obstructive jaundice. The tumor exhibits differentiation in different cell types including epithelioid cells in nests and trabeculae, spindle cells in fascicles and scattered ganglion cells. It will variously stain with chromogranin A, synaptophysin, NSE, somatostatin and pancreatic peptide hormones.

The Gangliocytic paragangliomas behave in a benign fashion but lymph node metastasis is encountered in few cases. A recent large epidemiological survey of 192 GP cases published in literature worldwide has produced valuable data, which is as follows: in 173 of 192 (69%) the tumor involved duodenum and lymph node metastasis was found in 12 of 173 (6.9%) cases. The tumor was larger in size and occurred in younger patients with lymph node metastasis (118, 119,120)

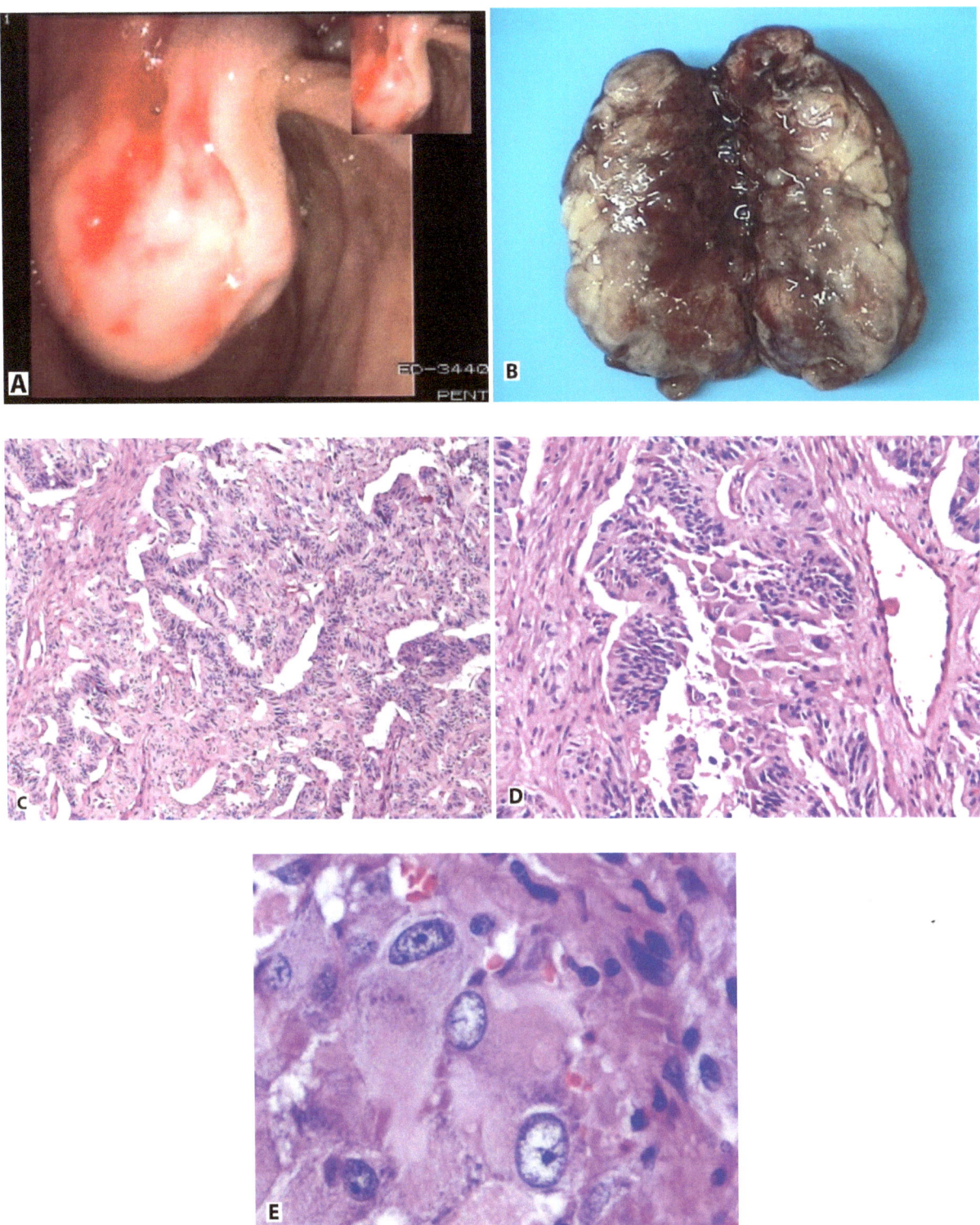

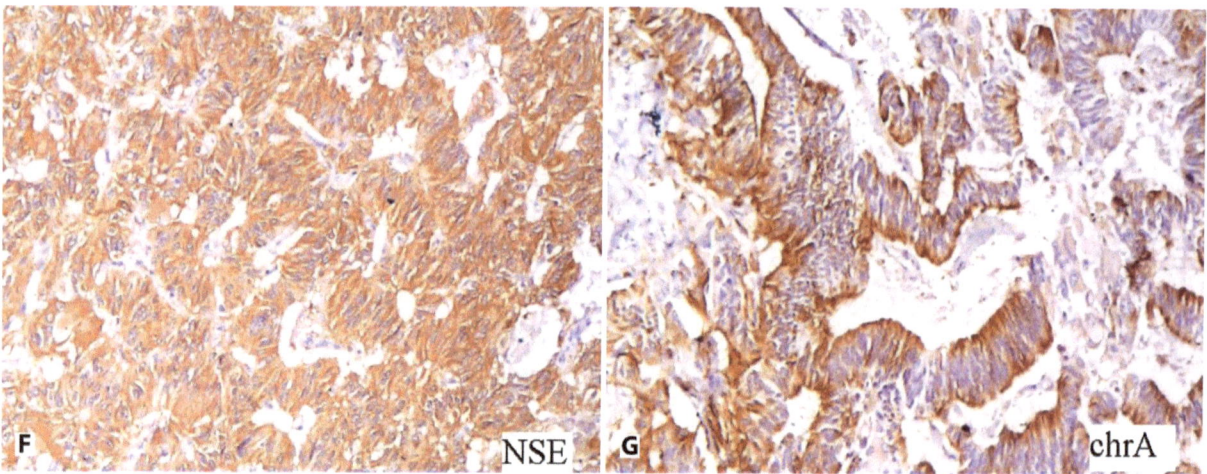

Figure 3.4 Gangliocytic Paraganglioma (A) smooth polypoid mass on endoscopy; (B) bisected tumor, (C, D) epithelioid and trabecular pattern (E) note large ganglion cells (F) strongly positive NSE (G) chromogranin focal strong staining. (Curtsey Dr Anita Shah, Pathologist Breach Candy Hospital)

Jejunal/Ileal Neuroendocrine tumors

NETs in jejunum and ileum are the most common (42%) among all GI NETs and at the time of clinical diagnosis the tumors were larger than 2 cm and showed transmural infiltration and metastasis in lymph nodes and liver.

Clinical Findings

Abdominal pain, nausea, vomiting and weight loss are the most frequent presenting symptoms. Signs of intestinal obstruction occur in some cases, usually secondary to ischemia related fibrosis and elastosis in the adventitia along with marked narrowing of medium sized vessels. Not uncommonly, diagnosis of small bowel NET is made because of the presence of carcinoid syndrome with elevated levels of serum 5 HIAA. Serotonin producing tumors constitute most of the small bowel carcinoids and majority of carcinoid syndrome cases arise in small bowel.

Pathological Features

Small intestinal NETs occur as firm nodules just below the mucosal surface or within intestinal wall or bulge into mucosa. The size varies from 1 to 2 cm and can be as large as 3.5 cm. It appears pale brown or tan yellow on cut section. Histologically, the tumor cells appear small round or cuboidal forming nests separated by delicate vascular strands. The nuclei have fine stippled chromatin and indistinct nucleoli. A trabecular or acinar pattern may be encountered. There is a variable desmoplasia, often quite marked with sclerosing elastotic change in adventitia and intima of medium sized mesenteric arteries. Fibrosis involves muscle and serosa, which can cause kinking of the bowel loop leading to obstruction. Local lymph nodes are involved early and metastatic tumor bearing nodes may be larger than the primary growth. Hepatic metastases are common and can be quite massive, which may be the presenting feature without known prior intestinal carcinoid.

Prognosis

At the time of the clinical diagnosis, 60% of small intestinal carcinoids show metastasis to nodes. Even a small sized (<1 cm) NET can metastasize and cause death. Hence, small intestinal carcinoid is to be considered a potentially malignant lesion. However, these tumors exhibit a characteristic slow indolent growth and 5 year survival of 40% to 58% is far better than 5% survival rate of stage matched adenocarcinoma. A long term survival in patients with hepatic metastases has been reported. In a study of 167 jejunal-ileal 121 NETs 5% had carcinoid syndrome, 26% were multiple, 77% murally invasive, 31% had nodal metastasis and 5 year survival was 58% (121). In the last 3 decades no change has been seen in the mortality of ileal carcinoids (122,123). The salient points about diagnosis of malignant carcinoid tumor include cellular pleomorphism, size >2 cm, irregular hyperchromatic nuclei, frequent mitotic activity, necrosis, invasion muscularis mucosae.

Colonic Neuroendocrine Tumor

(Recto-sigmoid and Appendix excluded)

Majority of colonic NETs arise from, enterochromaffin cells and a few are undifferentiated small cell carcinomas similar to "oat" cell carcinoma of lung, Colonic carcinoids are the most aggressive and clinically present with abdominal mass, weight loss and dyspeptic symptoms.

At surgery the tumors are found to be large, bulky and invasive. Only 5% of these cases exhibit carcinoid syndrome and 65% occur in cecum and right colon. In an epidemiological study of 279 cases 203 were colonic and 76 ileo-cecal carcinoid tumors. The characteristic features included high incidence in females, cecum very commonly involved, 90% cases had >2 cm tumor size, delay in detection of right colonic site tumors, 61% with metastases at detection and 5 year survival about 40%. The 5- year survival rate was only 25% for those with distant spread. (124,125,126,127)

Recto-sigmoid Neuroendocrine Tumor

Rectal carcinoids account for 27% of all GI carcinoids. In a recent series, carcinoids of midgut (cecum to transverse colon) represented about 8% and those of hindgut (descending colon to recto-sigmoid) 20% of total 5973 gastrointestinal carcinoids. It is a slow growing tumor with a low incidence (14%) of lymph node metastasis. Rectal carcinoids are almost never associated with the carcinoid syndrome. The lesion is a sessile polyp or a small (<1 cm) nodule with yellowish cut surface and located in the mid-portion of the rectum. About 50% of rectal carcinoids are asymptomatic and discovered on rectal examination and endoscopy. The remaining 50% give rise to rectal bleeding, pain and constipation. Rectal carcinoids secrete a variety of peptide hormones including enteroglucagon (glycentin), PYY and pancreatic polypeptide. However, unlike other carcinoids rectal NET does not secrete chromogranin A but in its place chromogranin B is identified immunohistochemically. Whereas, a vast majority of these carcinoids are adequately treated with local excision radical surgery is carried out in case of large sized (>2 cm) tumor with muscle invasion, necrosis and high mitotic rate. The 5 year survival is a robust 88% and occurrence of invasion and metastasis is as low as 4%. In one study, malignant carcinoids accounted for 71% of colonic carcinoids and only 14% cases among rectal carcinoids. (128,129,130,131,132)

Appendicular Neuroendocrine Tumor

Most appendicular carcinoids are removed incidentally at laparotomy and some removed with a prior diagnosis of acute appendicitis. They are usually small, rarely metastasize and usually do not give rise to carcinoid syndrome. A few may behave in a malignant fashion and this is often apparent at laparotomy. There are three major histological types of neuroendocrine tumors: conventional EC cell tumor, goblet cell carcinoid and L-cell NET. Of these, EC cell tumor is the most frequent and well-studied NET, 70% occurring at the tip (Figure. 3.5 A-D) and 20% in the mid portion. They are pale yellow colored <1 cm nodules typically arising from the submucosa, although invasion in muscularis and lymphatics is quite common. (123,134,135)

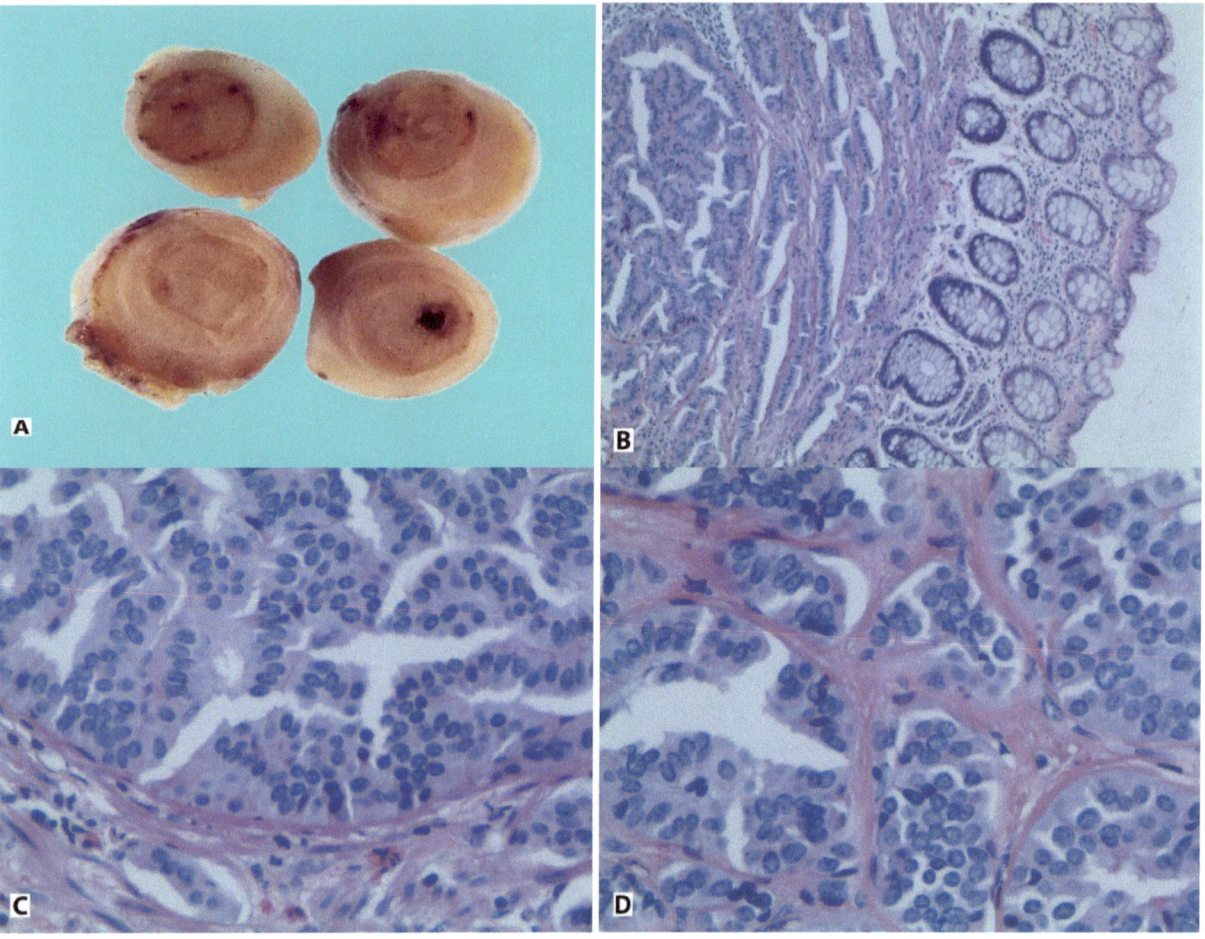

Figure 3.5 Carcinoid of appendix: (A) transverse section of thick swollen appendix plugged with pale tan yellowish tumor (B) intact appendicular mucosa overlying the tumor having trabecular pattern (C, D) small, uniform oval to round nuclei without anaplasia

Goblet cell carcinoid involves the appendix almost exclusively and the term goblet cell carcinoid has many synonyms: adenocarcinoid, mucinous carcinoid, crypt cell carcinoid and mucin producing neuroendocrine tumor.

This unique tumor arises from pluripotent crypt-base stem cells and shows dual differentiation, neuroendocrine and mucinous. Goblet cell carcinoid (GCC) is composed of mixture of normal crypt cells, goblet cells, Paneth cells and also enterochromaffin cells. The histological hallmark is the presence of clusters of goblet cells in the lamina propria or submucosa, and stain with neuroendocrine markers with patchy intensity (Figure 3.6 A, B, C). The tumor typically shows glandular collections of cells distended with mucous giving resemblance to goblet cells or signet ring cells (Figure. 3.6 A). Endocrine cells are sparsely populated and typically contain small peripheral nuclei with no pleomorphism and no mitotic activity. Size of the tumor and perineural lymphatic spread are unreliable prognostic features in GCC.

The prognosis of GCC is intermediate between appendicular carcinoid and pure appendicular adenocarcinoma. However, a subset of GCC is particularly aggressive. These reveal a mixture of conventional goblet cell carcinoid and foci of pure adenocarcinoma or typical signet ring cells with prominent nuclear anaplasia. The goblet cell carcinoid is known to metastasize to the ovary with no clinical evidence of appendiceal tumor. The ovarian tumor is often bilateral and is diagnosed as primary mucinous tumors of ovary (136,137,138,139).

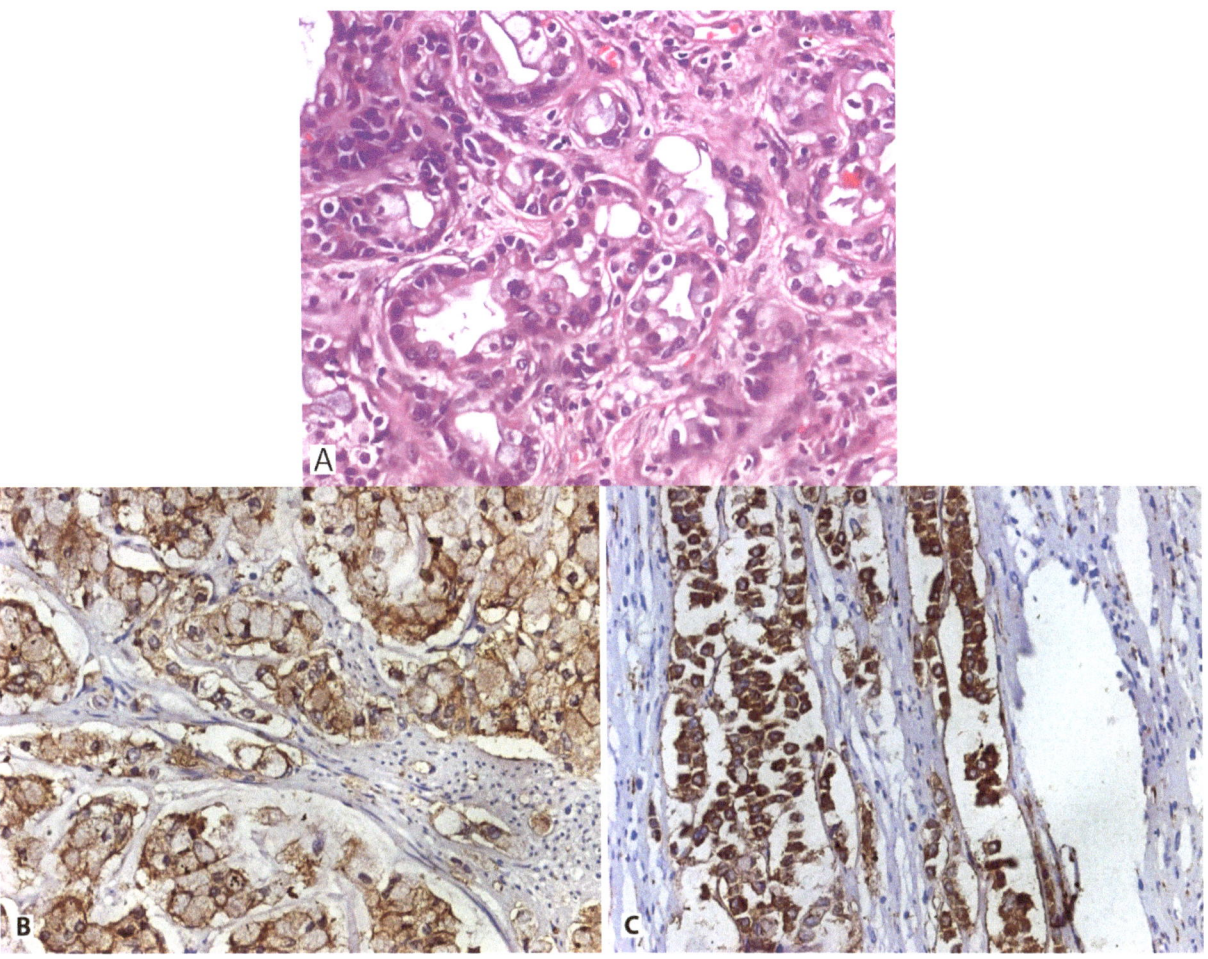

Figure 3.6 Goblet cell carcinoid (A) many cuboidal cells filled mucin and scattered small round cells (B) synaptophysin staining the mucinous cells (C) synaptophysin staining the small cell component

L-cell NET of Appendix

This type of NET is quite uncommon, very small (2-3 mm) in size and express enteroglucagon, PYY and pancreatic polypeptide but no chromogranin A. They are composed of small acini or tubules dispersed in loose fibrous stroma. The prognosis is good and some believe that they may not be truly neoplastic and represent a reactive change (135).

Treatment

Simple appendectomy is adequate and curative for appendiceal carcinoid <1 cm. For tumors 1-2 cm a simple appendectomy followed by periodic follow up for 5 years is recommended. Right hemicolectomy, 3 months after appendectomy, should be reserved for tumors >2 cm, tumor at the base of appendix, cecal infiltration, invasion into mesoappendix and associated adenocarcinoma.(140)

Pancreatic Endocrine Tumors (PETs):

General Considerations

(141,142,143,144)

A variety of functionally active endocrine tumors occurs in pancreas and these give rise to very dramatic signs and symptoms, which are typical of many clinical syndromes. All pancreatic endocrine tumors secrete a multitude of peptic hormones and amines, which cause clinical syndromes: insulin syndrome, glucagonoma syndrome, Zollinger-Ellison syndrome {excess gastrin secretions), VIPOMAS and WHDA (vomiting, diarrhea, hypocalcemia and achlorhydria). This has been also called as Verner-Morrison syndrome. The tumors are quite uncommon but their incidence has been increasing in the recent years. This is apparently due to application of more sensitive diagnostic approaches such as: imaging techniques, reliable laboratory tests and analysis by immunohistochemical and molecular biology assays. The relative incidence of PETs from the WHO data is given in Table 3.7. Tables 3.8, 3.9 show the author's experience of various pancreatic lesions, including the list of 21 endocrine tumors (incidence 2.3%).

Pancreatic Endocrine Tumors

(WHO data: n=638, Heitz PU, Bordi C, Komminath P,et al. WHO classification of Tumors, Pathology and Genetics : Tumors of Endocrine Organs. Delellis PA, Lloyd RV, Heitz PU, Eng C (Eds) IARC press Lyon, 2004) 143

Table 3.7 : Pancreatic Endocrine Tumors[143] (WHO data: n=638)*	
Insulinomas	174(27.2%)
Gastrinomas	80(12.5%)
Glucagonomas	51 (8%)
VIPomas	41 (6.4%) 24
Somatostatinoma	24 (3.80%)
Ectopic hormone tumors	15(2.4%
Nonfunctioning	253 (39.7%)

Table 3.8: Lesions of Pancreas, n=895 Author's series (1970-2000)	
Adenocarcinoma of pancreas	157
Adenocarcinoma of ampulla	110
Adenoma, cystadenoma	9
Endocrine tumors	21
Non-neoplastic lesions	598
Total	895

Table 3.9: Endocrine tumors of pancreas Author's seris (1970-2000) n=21	
Benign Insulinoma	8
Malignant Insulinoma	2
Malignant Gastrinoma	2
Stomatostatinoma	1
Glucagonoma	1
Carcinoid with syndrome	1
Nonfunctiomng, Benign	4
Nonfunctiomng, malignant	2

Histology:

Most PETs are well differentiated and have different morphological patterns, namely: trabecular, solid, glandular, gyriform, etc. The cells are small to medium sized with pale cytoplasm and finely distributed chromatin ("salt & pepper" nuclei). All features area sufficiently distinctive to permit identification of endocrine nature of a given tumor. In general, histological pattern is not specific for different syndromic tumors and the diagnosis in most instances is made before surgery. There are two exceptions to this rule: amyloid deposit in the tumor is indicative of insulinoma and glandular structures with psammoma bodies are commonly observed in somatostatinoma.

Prediction of the behavior of PETs

The behavior of PETs is difficult to predict on their histological features alone. Metastasis is generally accepted to be the only definitive feature of malignancy. However, several characteristics such as tumor size, presence and type of hyper functioning syndrome, number of mitoses, Ki 67 Proliferative Index, vascular/perineural invasion, necrosis and grade of tumor have been reported as reliable prognostic markers. Multivariate approaches, such as Capella (144) classification combine some of these parameters to group PETs into four subgroups: benign, borderline, low grade malignant and high grade malignant. This classification is based on tumor size, histologic parameters, including tumor differentiation, vascular invasion and functional lineage.

Facts:

- Insulinomas and nonfunctional noninvasive well differentiated PETs less than 2 cm size usually behave benign.
- Insulinomas and nonfunctional tumors greater than 3 cm and /or angioinvasive tumors are generally classified as low grade malignant PETs.
- Noninvasive tumors between 2cm and 3cm form a group whose behavior is difficult to predict and are designated as "borderline".
- Gastrinoma, VIPoma, glucagonoma, or tumors with Cushing or carcinoid syndromes with >2 cm size and/or angioinvasion are classified as low grade malignant, those less than 1 cm as benign, those between 1 cm and 2 cm as borderline.
- Tumors histologically resembling small cell adenocarcinomas constitute the poorly differentiated endocrine carcinomas.

Recently Cytokeratin 19 has been shown to be a powerful predictor of survival in pancreatic endocrine tumors. The authors of this article suggested that all PETs with any one of the following features be diagnosed as malignant: presence of necrosis, vascular invasion, perineurial invasion or CK 19 positivity. It is necessary to stain endothelial cells by immunohistochemical marker CD34 to identify small vascular channels, not clearly evident on H & E stain.

Neurofibromatosis & PETs

It is well known that patients with von Recklinghausen syndrome (NF1) are predisposed to endocrine tumors including pheochromocytoma and duodenal neuroendocrine tumors (carcinoids) secreting somatostatin. It is not known whether rarely occurring insulinoma in VRS is an incidental finding or whether it is a rare manifestation of NF1.

Insulinoma, glucagonoma, Gastrinoma and Somatostatinoma will be described and illustrated.

Insulinoma

(146, 147, 148)

This is insulin secreting common benign endocrine tumor of the Beta cells of islets of Langerhans, giving rise to sustained intractable hypoglycemia before surgical intervention. A vast majority of insulinomas are located in the pancreas and less than 2% in the duodenal wall. The tumors are almost equally distributed in head, body and tail of the pancreas. Determination of plasma insulin and proinsulin concentration by radioimmunoassay has greatly facilitated the diagnosis. Grossly, the tumor is well circumscribed or encapsulated and the malignant ones appear nodular. Microscopic study shows four types of patterns, the most common being trabecular. The cells frequently show bland cytology with no nuclear anaplasia (Figure. 3.7 A-E). One of the most characteristic finding in insulinoma is amyloid stroma. (Figure. 3.7 F, G). Histopathologic study is required mainly to confirm benignancy, which is present in 95% of cases and to look for signs of malignancy such as local invasion and metastasis. Malignant insulinomas may show invasion in the peripancreatic tissue or adjacent organs, and metastases to regional lymph nodes (peripancreatic, celiac and paraaortic) and liver.

The natural history and survival:

A study of 1067 cases of Insulinoma **(Stephanini P, Carboni M, Pathrossi N, et al. Beta islet cell tumors of the pancreas: results of a study of 1067 cases. Surgery 1974; 75:597-609)** [147]

638/1012 (63%) completely documented cases were reported to be all cured. In 772 (76%) cases tumor was found at operation. In 74 (7%) cases no tumor was found at operation. Second operation was required in 111 (11%) cases, multiple operations were required in 58 (5.7%) cases. The distribution of tumors was as follows: head (305), body (285) & tail (323). In 789 (83%) cases single tumor present, in 123 (13%) cases multiple tumors present and 39 (4%) cases were associated with MEN 1. Different types of surgeries included: enucleation 506 (50%), distal resection 415(41%), subtotal resection 20 (2%) and pancreatico-duodenectomy 15 (1.5%)

Service FJ, McMahon MM, Obstriet PC, et al Functioning insulinoma: incidence, recurrences and long term survival of patients, 60 year study Mayo Clin Proc 1991; 66:711-719) [148]

Median age in this study was 47 yrs. in males and 59 yrs. in females. Recurrence rate associated with MEN1 was 21% at 10-20 years in contrast to 5% recurrence rate associated with sporadic cases at 10 years & 7% at 20 years. The 10 year survival in cases of benign Insulinoma was 88% vs 29% in cases of malignant insulinomas.

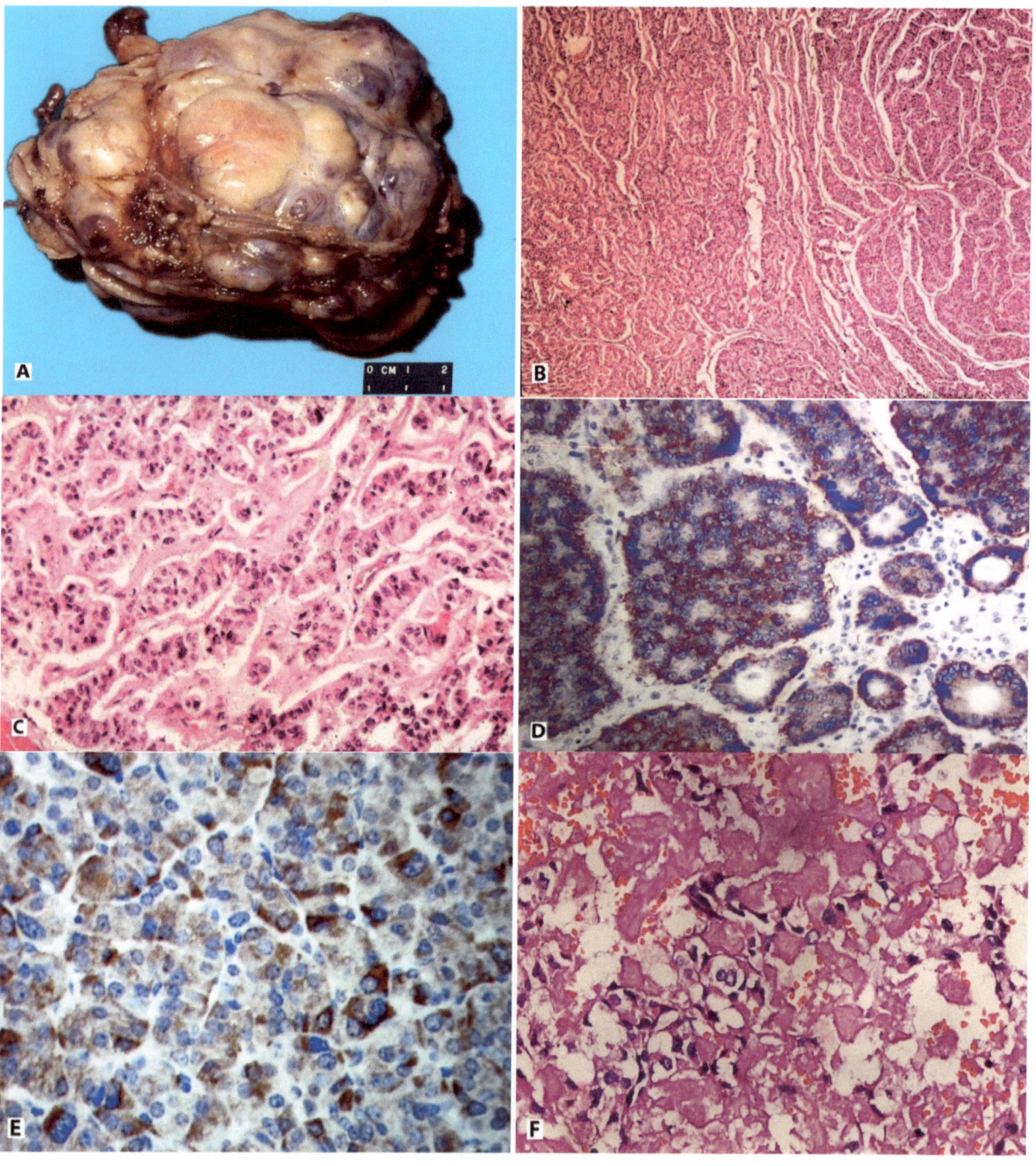

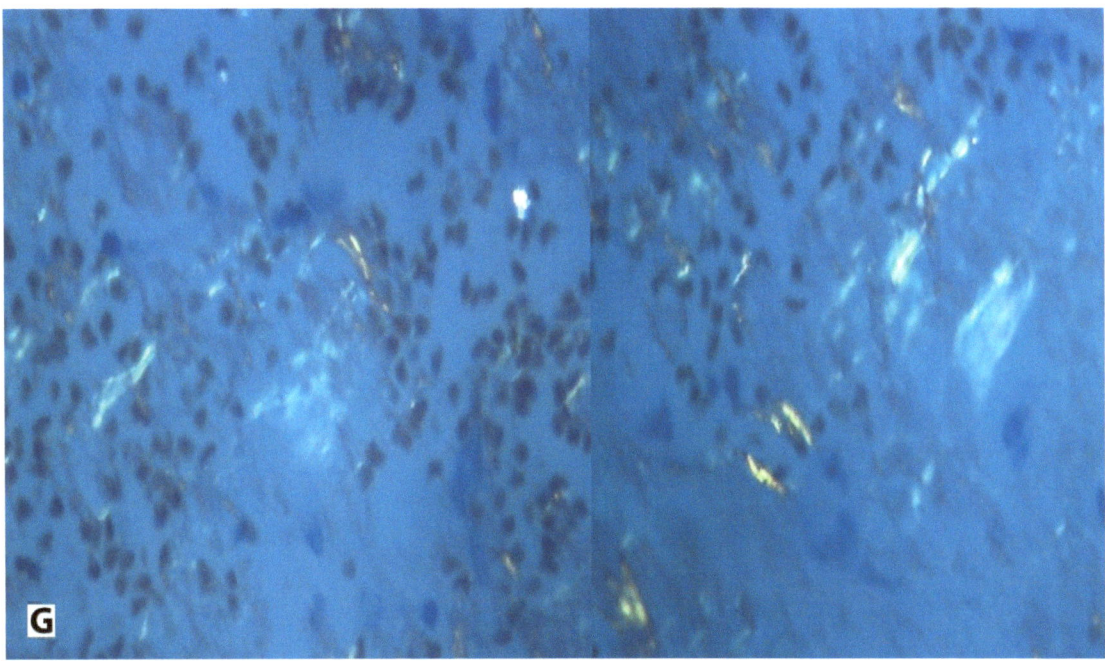

Figure 3.7 Insulinoma of pancreas: (A) nonfunctioning Insulinoma is a bosselated well encapsulated 11 x 8 x 5 cm mass, (B& C) trabecular pattern; variable nuclear anaplasia (D) glandular pattern (E) tumor cells express insulin on immunohistochemistry (F) histology of amyloid stroma in insulinoma (G) Cong red stain showing focal green fluorescence on polarized light

Glucagonoma

Glucagonoma syndrome is a paraneoplastic phenomenon characterized by islet alpha-cell pancreatic tumor, necrolytic migratory erythema, diabetes mellitus, weight loss, anemia, stomatitis, thromboembolism, gastrointestinal disturbances and neuropsychiatric symptoms. The frequency of each of these presenting signs is shown in Table 3.10. These findings in association with hyperglucagonemia and demonstrable pancreatic tumor establish the diagnosis. Most patients are diagnosed too late in the clinical course for cure but successful palliation of symptomatology can usually be achieved. Glucagonoma associated with MEN 1 syndrome tend to be multiple in about 59% of cases. Majority of glucagonoma are large solitary tumors with a 7 cm mean diameter (Figure. 3.8 A-C). The histological features are not distinctive in any way and the diagnosis is often suggested by a set of presenting symptoms confirmed by demonstration of hyperglucagonemia.

The tumors spread by local invasion into surrounding tissues and metastasize to regional nodes and liver. About 60 % to 70% glucagonomas present with metastasis at the time of diagnosis. Even small sized (<0.5 cm) glucagonomas are known to show uncertain behavior or a histologically identified well differentiated endocrine carcinoma. (149,150)

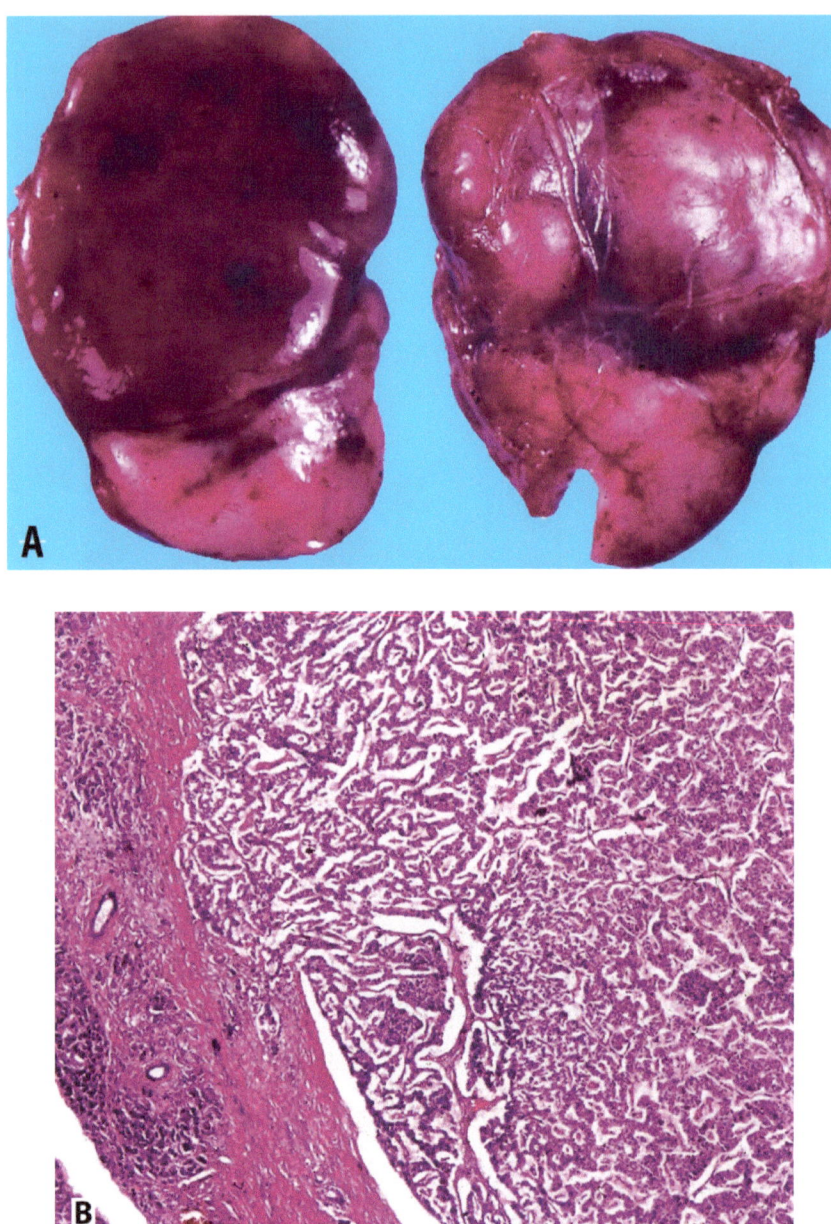

Figure 3.8 Glucagonoma: (A) encapsulated bosselated functioning glucagonoma (B) trabecular pattern of neoplastic endocrine cells and the tumor invading the thick fibrous capsule

GASTRO-ENTERO-PANCREATIC ENDOCRINE TUMORS

Table 3.10 Clinical features of glucagonomas-407 cases[150]	
Associated with MEN1	53/407 (13%)
Incidence of multiple tumors	48/407 (12%)
Situated in tail of pancreas	213/407 (54%)
Malignancy	247/407 (61%)
Metastases	209/407 (51%)
Patients with Diabetico-dermatogenic Syndrome (DDS)	233/407 (57%)
10yr survival in 233 cases with DDS	with metastasis-52%
	without metastasis 64%

Gastrinoma

Gastrinomas are gastrin producing endocrine tumors that occur almost exclusively in pancreatico-duodenal region. Most are functional, causing hypergastrinemia and Zollinger Ellison syndrome (ZES). This syndrome is characterized by multiple duodenal peptic ulcers prominent gastric rugal folds secondary to an increased oxyntic gland mass, and steatorrhoea. Two types of gastrinomas occur: sporadic non familial gastrinoma with ZES (80% of cases) and familial gastrinoma with ZES in the setting of MEN 1 (20% of cases). Gastrinomas are relatively common functioning endocrine tumors of pancreas and duodenum and are second in frequency only to insulinomas.

Location of gastrinomas is much more common in pancreas (53%) than in duodenum or jejunum (13%) according to the data of ZES tumor registry with 800 cases as of 1973 (151).

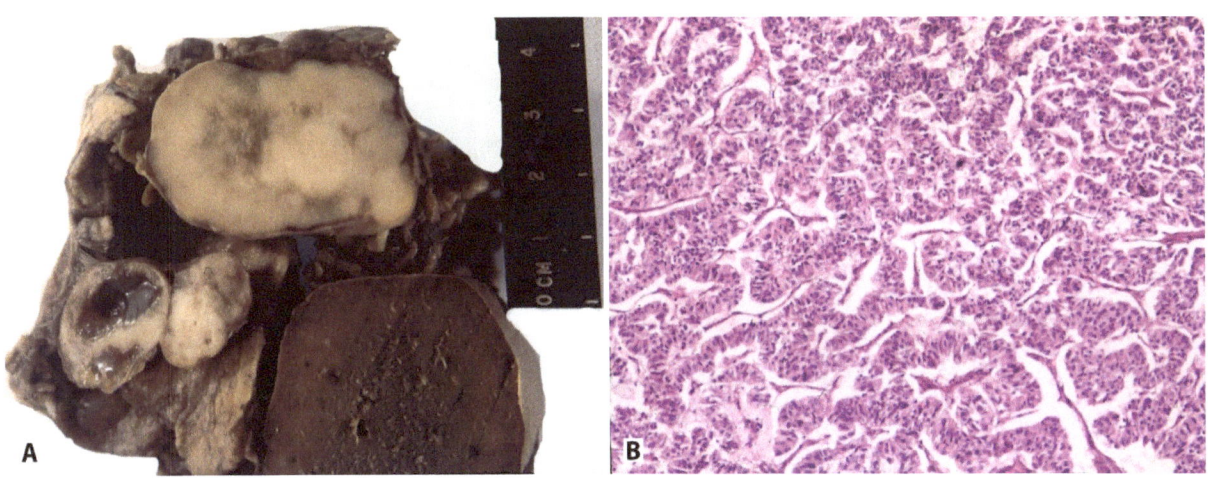

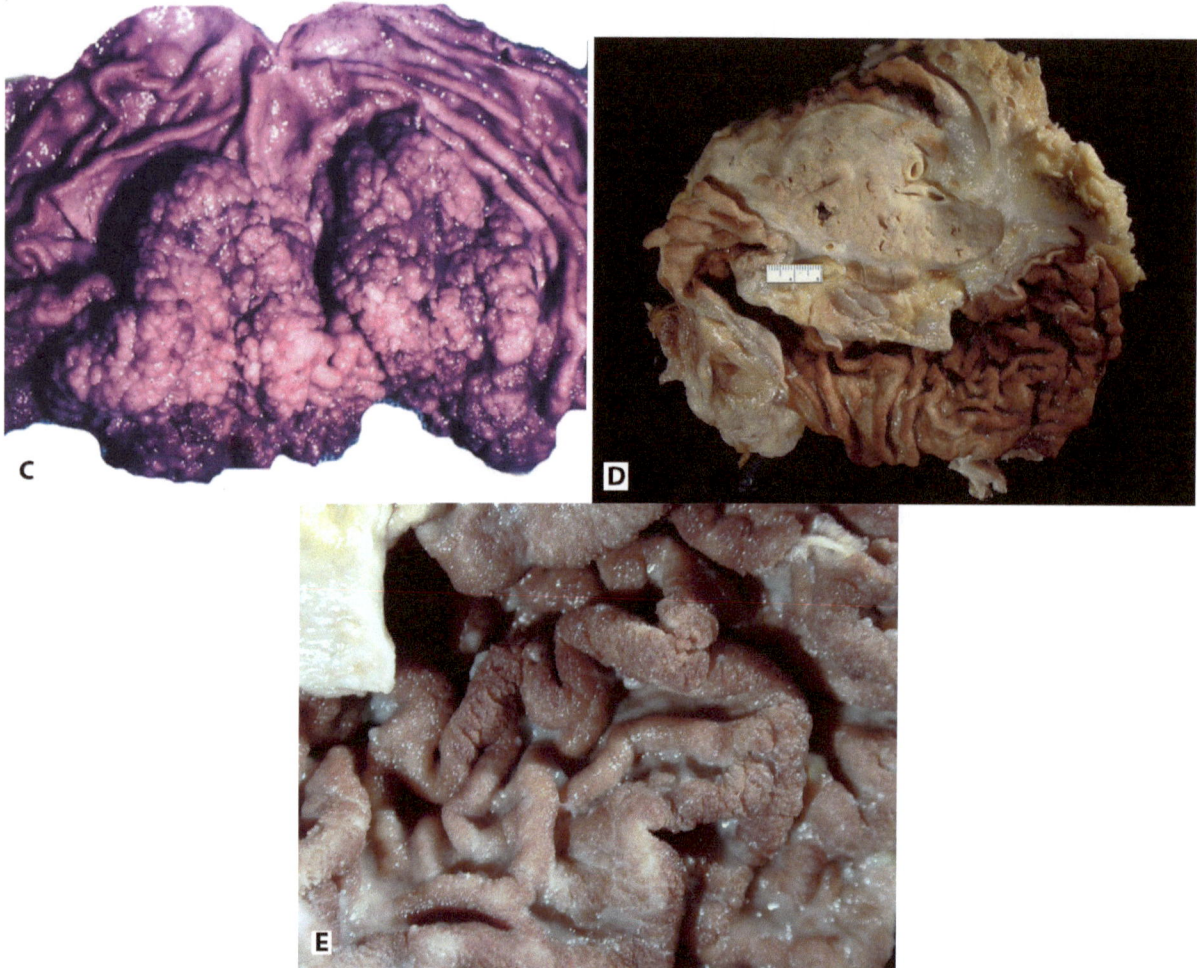

Figure 3.9 Zollinger–Ellison syndrome: (A) A large 6 cm encapsulated tumor with satellite nodules and spleen with stomach in the background (B) typical trabecular pattern of a cellular lesion (C) gastric mucosal folds (rugae) enormously thickened due to florid hyperplasia of parietal cells superficially resembling a neoplasm, no adenoma, was found. (D) ill-defined tumor in pancreas adherent to stomach (E) hypertrophic gastric mucosal rugae

Gastrinoma are usually residing within "gastrinoma triangle", which is formed by junction of cystic duct and common duct, the junction of II and III parts of duodenum and junction of neck and body of the pancreas. It is extraordinary that gastrinoma has been reported in far flung organ systems including stomach, biliary tract, liver, kidney, mesentery and heart.

Gastrinomas are cellular tumors (Figure. 3.9 A-F) composed of anastomosing cords, trabeculae and lobules lined by monotonous cells with eosinophilic cytoplasm and round nuclei having fine chromatin. Both sporadic gastrinomas and those associated with the setting of MEN 1 may be multifocal. Multiple sporadic gastrinomas probably represent metastasis, because all independent tumors share identical mutations and other genetic changes. Those associated with MEN 1 have varied genetic abnormalities and probably represent independent primary tumors. It is important to distinguish gastrinomas from other type of PETs because gastrinoma diagnosis has far reaching clinical implications. Incidentally discovered duodenal lesions associated with chronic acid suppression or gastritis, behave in a clinically indolent fashion and should be treated conservatively. Peripancreatic and periduodenal gastrinomas are thought to represent primary tumors rather than metastases from an occult primary in the duodenum. Some patients have been cured after resection of the tumorous nodes.

Treatment & Prognosis

Management of ZES is a formidable problem because of dreadful consequences of acid overproduction, difficulty in localizing of gastrinoma particularly in the duodenum (often small sized), multiple tumors and overall poor survival. The use of powerful acid anti secretory agents like H2 receptor antagonist and proton pump inhibitors has profoundly facilitated management of ZES. In the past patients with ZES were treated with total gastrectomy but now the care is primarily focused on management of the gastrinoma tumor (152, 153).

In a series of 52 cases of ZES a search for gastrinomas was carried out at exploratory laparotomy. **The study gives a wealth of information about the role of surgery in the management and its effects on prognosis** (152).

- Gastrinoma involves the entire pancreas in most patients with MEN 1
- Total pancreatectomy may be necessary to cure ZES in MEN 1
- It is possible to cure some patients with hepatic metastases
- Tumors of the head of pancreas can be cured by enucleation alone
- The morbidity of operations aimed at removing all gastrinoma is very low today.
- Resections of all visible gastrinomas in patient without MEN have about 70% chance of curing the patient.
- The quality of life after successful surgery is so much better than other forms of therapy that possibility of resection should be aggressively pursued in every patient

Gastrinoma in patients with liver metastasis behave more aggressively (153) than those with only lymph node metastasis. In fact lymph node metastases have little or no influence on the survival on patients with ZES (154). The frequency of metastasis is 30% in patients with pancreatic gastrinoma and only 3% in patients with duodenal tumors. Metastases to other organs are indeed rare. It has been observed that duodenal gastrinomas are less malignant (38%) than pancreatic ones (60%). In general progression of gastrinomas is relatively slow with a combined 5-year survival of 65% and 10-year survival of 51%. Even with metastatic disease a 10-year survival for lymph node metastases is 46% and for liver metastases 40%. In patients with complete resection have excellent 5 and 10-year survival rates of 90-100%. Patients with pancreatic tumors have a worst prognosis than those with duodenal tumor: 10-year survival of 9% versus 59%. The rate of death in aggressive forms of gastrinoma ranges from 38% in MEN 1 cases to 62% in sporadic cases. (155,156,157,158)

Nesidioblastosis

(158,159,160)

Hyperinsulinism is a rare cause of severe persistent hypoglycemia during the neonatal period. Nevertheless it is a diagnosis of importance since hypoglycemia may be exceedingly difficult to control. The patient should undergo a subtotal pancreatectomy as soon as the diagnosis is reached because of high incidence of brain damage and subsequent mental retardation. The syndrome was described more than 40 years ago but the pathogenesis of the disease has not yet been completely elucidated. The term nesidioblastosis describes the persistence of a diffused disseminated proliferation of islets cells budding off from ducts (ducto-insulinar complex) Electron microscopic study is diagnostic of Nesidioblastosis, in that the characteristic crystalline granules of beta cells can be readily differentiated from zymogen granules (Figures 3.10, 3.11) This excess mass of beta cells is considered to be the underlying cause of the disease. However, it has been seen that nesidioblastosis is encountered in the pancreas in normo-glycemic neonates and infants, which was observed at autopsy. This implies that pathogenesis of nesidioblastosis should be reconsidered and other causative factors be investigated. By means of linkage analysis, hyperinsulinism in familial cases has been shown to chromosome 11 and ongoing genetic studies await the elucidation of the pathogenesis of nesidioblastosis.

Nesidioblastosis is also an infrequent, yet clinically important, cause of hypoglycemia in adult population, and should be considered in a patient with a presumptive diagnosis of insulinoma. A 70% distal pancreatectomy will be successful in controlling hyperglycemia in these patients, and would rarely result in diabetes mellitus (161)

A case of hyperinsulinimic hypoglycemic coma in a 1 year old child is illustrated in (Figures 3.10 & 3.11).

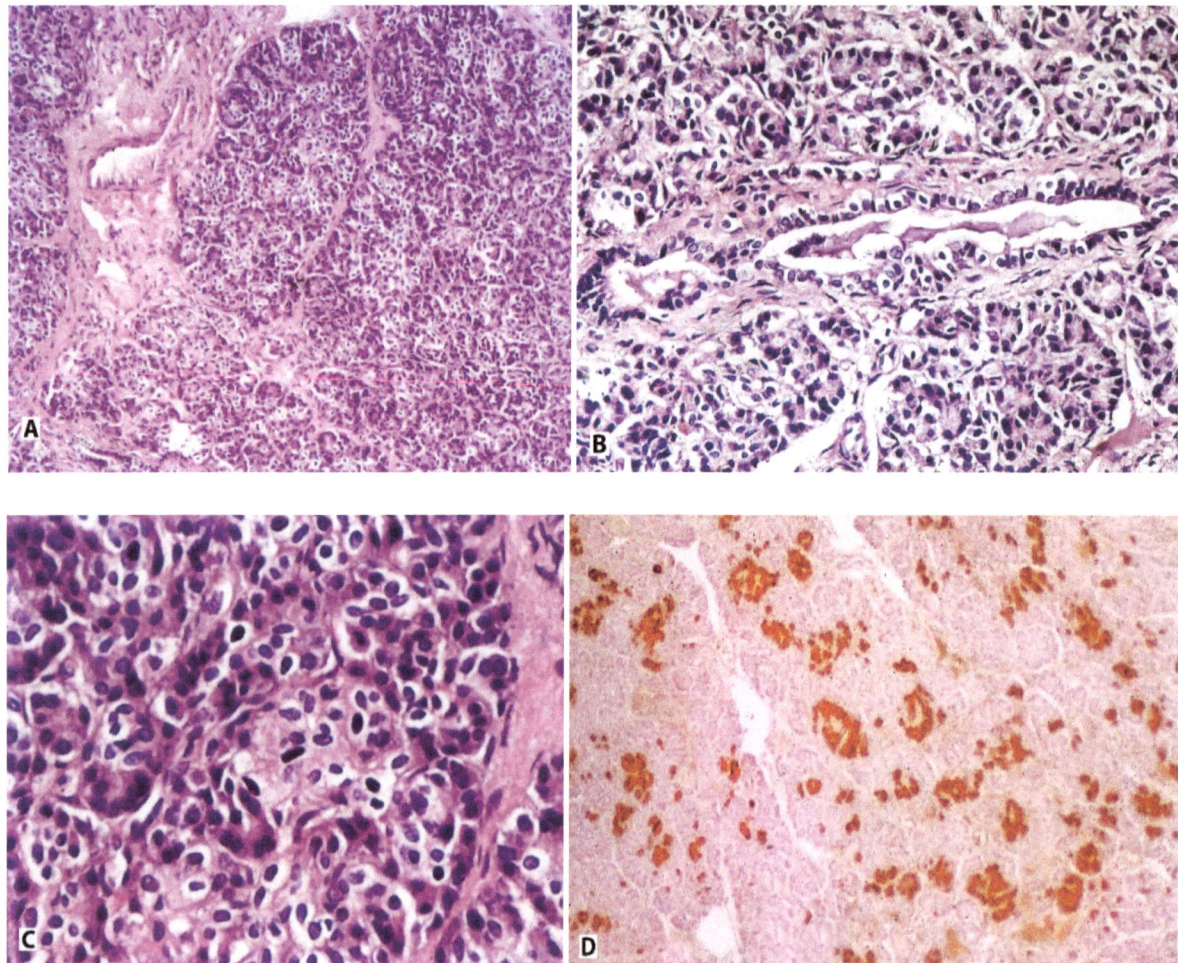

Figure 3.10 Nesidioblastosis (A) Section of pancreas exhibiting a large population of vacuolated cells (endocrine cells)within the acini, note lack of islets (B) The vacuolated cells are also seen within the lining of pancreatic ducts (C) high power view of overwhelming number of larger vacuolated endocrine cells (D) Numerous small clusters of cells expressing insulin on immunohistochemistry

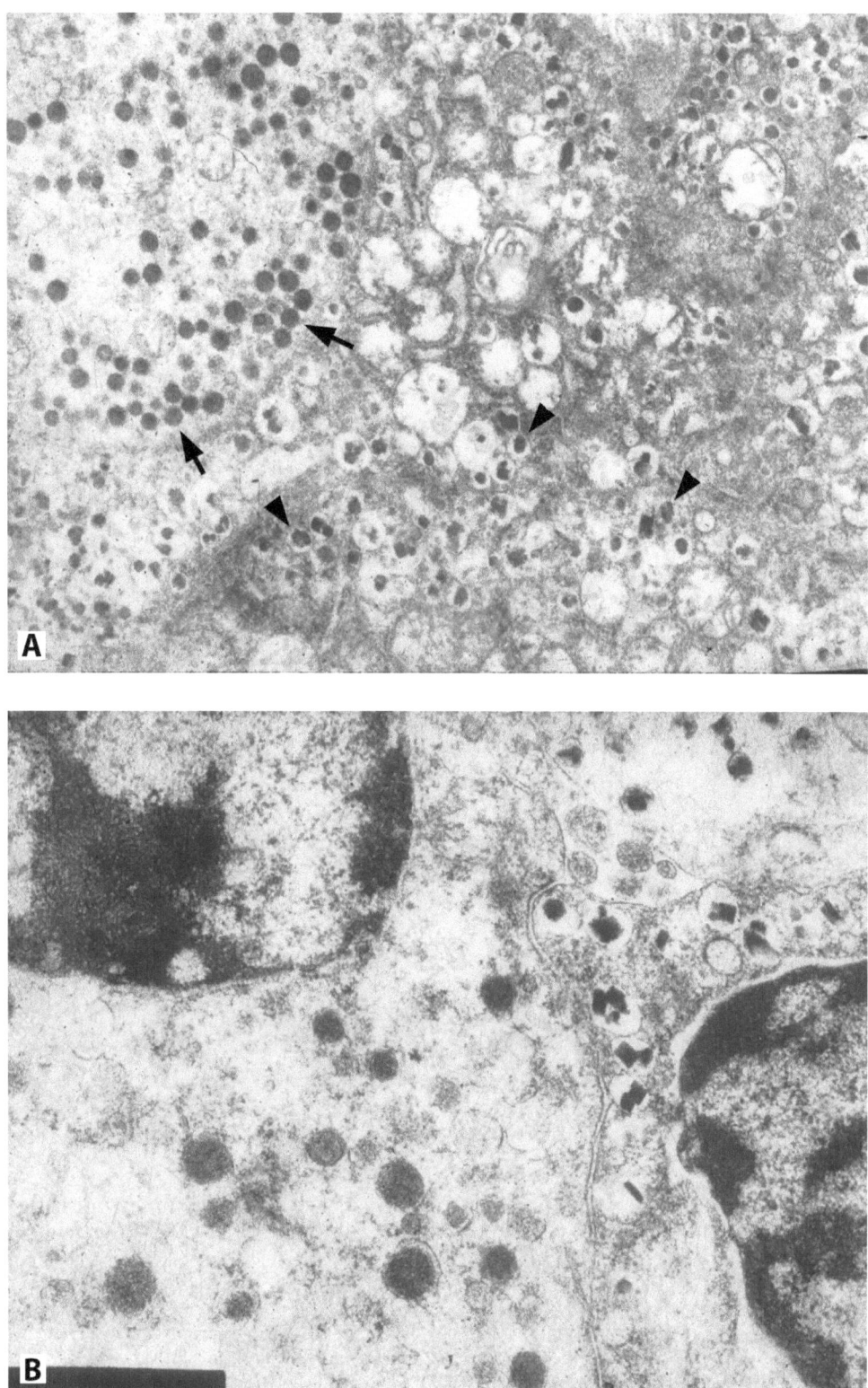

Figure 3.11 (A) Electron microscopy of nesidioblastosis of pancreas: numerous large rounded zymogen granules (black arrows) and irregular pleomorphic beta (insulin) granules (arrow heads)in the same cells (B) higher power shows two cells separated by double plasma membranes with rounded exocrine zymogen granules seen in cell on left and pleomorphic beta insulin granules in cell on right. This is in the same pancreatic acinus.

Refrences of Gastro-Entero-Pancreatic Neuroendocrine Tumors

99 Kloppel G. Oberndorfer and His Successors: From carcinoid to Neuroendocrine Carcinoma Endocr Pathol 2007; 18:141,

100 Lewin KJ. The endocrine cells of the gastrointestinal tract. The normal endocrine cells and their hyperplasias, Part I. In Sommers Sc, Rosen PP {eds}: Pathology Annual. Part I. Vol 21. Appleton-Century Crafts, East Norwalk, CT, 1986

101 Pearse AGE. The APUD cell concept and its implications in pathology In Sommers Sc {ed}: Pathology Annual. Vol 9. Appleton-Century Crafts/New York, 1974

102 Polak JM and Bloom SR. Neuropeptides of the Gut: A Newly Discovered Major Control System. World J Surg 1979; 3:393

103 Kloppel G, Perren A, Heitz PU: The Gastroenteropancreatic Neuroendocrine Cell System and Its Tumors: The WHO classification. Ann. N. Y. Acad. Sci 2004; 1014:13-27

104 Modlin IM, Lye KD, Kidd M: A 5-decade Analysis of 13,715 Carcinoid Tumors. Cancer 2003; 97: 934-959)

105 Rindi G, Bordi C, Rappel S, et al: Gastric carcinoids and neuroendocrine carcinomas: Pathogenesis, pathology and behavior. World J Surg 1996; 20: 168-172

106 Bordi C, D'Adda T, Azzoni C, et al: Hypergastrinemia and gastric enterochromaffin-like cases. Am J Surg Pathol 1995; 19(Suppl 1) S8-S19

107 Bordi C, D'Adda T, Azzoni C, Ferraro G: Pathogenesis of ECL tumors in humans. Yale J Biol Med. 2003; 71: 273-284)

108 Modlin IM, Lye KD, Kidd M: Carcinoid tumors of the stomach. Surg Oncol 2003; 12: 153-172

109 Modlin IM, Lawton GP, Miu K, et al: Patho-physiology of the fundic enterochromaffin-like{ECL} and gastric carcinoid tumors. Ann R Coll Surg Engl 1996; 78: 1330138

110 Merchant SH, Vanderjagt T, Lathrop S, Amin MB: Sporadic duodenal bulb gastrin-cell tumors: Association with Helicobacter Pylori gastritis and long term use of proton pump inhibitors. Am J Surg Pathol 2006; 30:1581-1587

111 Peghini PL, Annibale B, Azzoni C, et al : Effects of chronic hypergastrinemia on human enterochromaffin-like cells: insights from patients with sporadic gastrinomas. Gastroenterology; 2002:123: 68-85

112 Modlin IM, Lye KD, Kidd M: A 50 year analysis of 562 gastric carcinoids: Small tumor or larger problem? Am J Gastroenterol 2004; 99: 23-32

113 Weisberg J, de Matos LL, do Amaral Antonio Mader AM, et al: Neuroendocrine gastric carcinoma expressing somatostatin: A highly malignant rare tumor. World J Gastroenterol 2006; 12: 3944-3947

114 Nicau GC, Toubanakis C, Nikolau P, et al: Gastrinomas associated with MEN-1 syndrome. New insights for the diagnosis and management in a series of 11 patients Hepatogastroenterology 2005; 52: 1668-1676

115 Dayal Y, Tallberg KA, Nunnemacher G, et al: Duodenal carcinoids in patients with and without neurofibromatosis: A comparative study. Am J Surg Pathol 1986; 10: 348-357

116 Bombstein-Quevedo L, Gamboa-Dominguez A: Carcinoid tumors of duodenum and ampulla of Vater: A clinicopathological, immunohistochemical, and cell kinetic comparison. Hum Pathol 2001; 32: 1252-1256

117 Makhlout HR, Burke AP, Sobin LH: Carcinoid tumors of the ampulla of Vater: A comparison with duodenal carcinoid tumors Cancer 1999; 85: 1241-1249

118 Williams GT: Endocrine tumors of the gastrointestinal tract. Selected topics Histopathology 2007; 5030-41

119 Scheithauer BW, Nora FE, Lechago J, et al: Duodenal Gangliocytic paraganglioma: Clinico-pathologic and immunocytochemical study of 11 cases. Am J Clin Pathol 1986; 2086: 559-556

120 Okubo Y, Wakayama M, Nemoto T, et al: Literature survey on epidemiology and pathology of Gangliocytic paraganglioma. BMC Cancer 2011; 11: 187

121 Burke AP, Thomas RM, Elsayed AM, Sobin LH; Carcinoids of the jejunum and ileum: An immunohistochemical and clinicopathological study of 167 cases. Cancer 1997; 79: 1086-1093

122 Soga J: Early-stage carcinoids of the gastrointestinal tract; An analysis of 1914 reported cases. Cancer 2005; 103: 1587-1595

123 Modlin IM, Champaneria MC, Chen AK, Kidd M; A three decade analysis of 3,914 small intestinal neuroendocrine tumors: The rapid pace of no progress. Am J Gastroenterol 2007; 102: 1464-1473

124 Modlin IM, Kidd M, Latich I, et al: Current status of gastrointestinal carcinoids. Gastroenterology 2005; 128: 1717-1721

125 Spread C, Berkel H, Jewel L, et al: Colon carcinoid tumors: A population based study. Dis Colon Rectum 1994; 37:482-491

126 Soga J: Carcinoids of the colon and ileo-cecal region: A statistical evaluation of 363 cases collected from the literature J Exp Clin Cancer Res 1998; 17: 139-148

127 Federspiel BH, Burke AP, Sobin LH, Shekika KM: Rectal and colonic carcinoids:A clinicopathological study of 84 cases. Cancer 1990: 65: 135-140

128 Modlin IM, Sandor A: An analysis of 8305 cases of carcinoid tumors. Cancer 1997: 79: 813-829

129 Burke M, Shepherd N, Mann CV: Carcinoid tumors of rectum and anus. Brit J Surg 1987; 74: 358-361

130 Rosenberg JM, Welch JP: Carcinoid tumors of the colon. A study of 72 patients. Am J Surg; 1985; 149: 775-779

131 Stinner B, Kisker O, Zeilke A, Rothmund M: Surgical management for carcinoid tumors of small bowel,, appendix, colon & rectum. World J Surg 1996; 20: 183-188

132 Jetmore AB, Ray JE, Gathright IB, et al: Rectal carcinoids, the most frequent carcinoid tumor. Dis Colon Rectum 1992; 35: 717-725

133 Tchana-Sato V, Detry O, Polus M, et al: Carcinoid Tumor of the Appendix: A consecutive series from 1237 appendectomies. World J Gastroenterol 2006; 12:669-96701

134 Givi B, Pommeir SJ, Thompson AK, et al: Operative resection of carcinoid neoplasms in patients with liver metastases yields significantly better survival. Surgery 2006; 140: 891-897

135 Car NJ, Sobin LH: Neuroendocrine tumors of the appendix. Semin Diagn Pathol 2004; 21: 108-119

136 Toumpanakis C, Sstandish RA, Baishnab E, et al: Goblet cell carcinoid tumors (adenocarcinoid) of the appendix. Dis Colon Rectum 2007; 50: 315-322

137 Warkel RL, Cooper PH, Helwig EB. Adenocarcinoid, a mucin-producing carcinoid tumor of the appendix: a study of 39 cases. Cancer 1978; 42:2781–2793.

138 Tang LH, Shia J, Soslow RA, et al: Pathologic classification and clinical behavior of the spectrum of goblet cell carcinoid tumors of the appendix. Am J Surg Pathol. 2008;32: 429–1443.

139 Burke AP, Sobi LH, Federspiel BH, et al: Goblet cell carcinoids and related tumors of the vermiform appendix. Am J Clin Pathol 1990; 94: 27-35

140 Griniatsos J, Michail O: Appendiceal neuroendocrine tumors: Recent insights and clinical implications. World J Gastrointest Oncol 2110; 2: 192-196

141 Larson Li. Pancreatic endocrine tumors. Hum Pathol 1978; 9:401-426

142 Kloppel G, Heitz PU. Tumors of the endocrine pancreas in Fletcher CMD Diagnostic histopathology of Tumors, 2007: Volume 2, Third edition, Churchill Livingstone

143 Heitz PU, Bordi C, Komminath P,et al. WHO classification of Tumors, Pathology and Genetics : Tumors of Endocrine Organs. Delellis PA, Lloyd RV, Heitz PU, Eng C (Eds) IARC press Lyon, 2004

144 Capella C, Heitz PU, Hopfler H, et al. Revised classification of neuroendocrine tumors of lung, pancreas and gut Virchow Arch 1995; 425:547-560

145 Deshpande V, Castilla CFD, Muzikansky, et al. Cytokeratin 19 Is a Powerful Predictor of Survival in Pancreatic Endocrine Tumors. Am J Surg Pathol 2004; 28:11145-1153

146 Tong-Hua L, Tseng HC, Zhu Yu, et al Insulinoma: An immunocytochemical and morphological analysis of 95 cases. Cancer 1985; 56:1420-1429

147 Stephanini P, Carboni M, Pathrossi N, et al. Beta islet cell tumors of the pancreas: results of a study of 1067 cases. Surgery 1974; 75:597-609

148 Service FJ, McMahon MM, Obstriet PC, et al Functioning insulinoma: incidence, recurrences and long term survival of patients, 60 year study Mayo Clin Proc 1991; 66:711-719

149 Chastain MA. The glucagonoma syndrome: a review of its features and discussion of new perspective. Am J Med Sci 2001; 321:306-320

150 Soga J, Yakuwa Y. Glucagonomas/diabetic-dermatogenic Syndrome: a statistical evaluation of 407 reported cases. J Hepatobiliary Pancreat Surg 1998; 5:312-319

151 Solcia E, Capella C, Kloppel G. Tumors of pancreas 1997, 3rd edition, Armed Forces Institute of Pathology, Washington DC

152 Fox PS, Hofmann JW, Wilson SD, et al. Surgical management of the Zollinger-Ellison Syndrome Surg Clin North Am 1974; 54:395-407

153 Deveney CW, Deveney KE, Stark D, et al. Resection of Gastrinomas. Ann Surg 1983; 198:546-553

154 Delcore r Jr, Chenung LY, Freisen SR. Outcome of lymph node involvement in patient of Zollinger-Ellison syndrome Ann Surg 1988;208:291-298

155 Stabile BE, Passaro EJ. Benign and malignant gastrinoma. Am J Surg 1985; 149:144-150

156 Gibril F, Venzon VJ, Ojeaburu JV et el. Prospective study of the natural history of in patients with MEN 1: definition of an aggressive and a nonagressive form. J Clin Endocrinol and Metab 2001; 86:5782-5293

157 Imamura M, Kanda M, Takahashi K, et al Clinicopathological characteristics of duodenal microgastrinomas. World J Surg 1992; 16:703-709

158 Sutliff VE, Doppman JL, Gibril F, et al. Growth of newly diagnosed untreated metastatic gastrinomas and predictors of growth pattern J Clin Oncol 1997; 15: 2420-2431

159 Rahier J, Guiot Y, Sempoux C. Persistent hyperinsulinimic hypoglycemic: a heterogeneous syndrome unrelated to nesidioblastosis Arch Dis Child Fetal Neonatal Ed 2000; 82:F108-F112

160 Palladino AA, Stanley CA. Nesidioblastosis No Longer! It's All About Genetics. Editorial, J Clin Endocrinol % Metab 2011; 96:617-619

161 Whittles RM, Straus IF, Sugg SL, et al. Adult onset nesidioblastosis causing hypoglycemia, an important clinical entity and continuing treatment dilemma Arch Surg 2001; 136: 656-663

www.ingramcontent.com/pod-product-compliance
Lightning Source LLC
Chambersburg PA
CBHW042032150426
43200CB00002B/24